Prologue: Remembering the Source While Drinking Water, Never Forgetting the Original Aspiration

Three Books That Led Me to the Path of Medicine

Wiping away the dust of the years, I unlock the floodgates of memory. Although the past has faded, it can still be vividly recalled...

I was born in October 1949, a time of great transformation in Chinese history.

In 1967, the Cultural Revolution was in full swing. I was 18 years old, classified as one of the "children who could be educated," meaning I wasn't eligible to become a Red Guard, and I belonged to the group known as the "free-riders." Prior to this, I loved reading, but now, there were no books to read. Every day, apart from playing basketball, swimming, or practicing boxing, I had nothing to do. I couldn't continue my studies, nor could I work to support my family. As a 17 or 18-year-old young man staying at home, living off my parents' meager salaries, I felt an overwhelming sense of burden.

One day in June that year, I strolled into the Dongsi Xinhua Bookstore, which was very close to my home. I used to visit this bookstore frequently. At that time, the bookstore had few books available, other than Mao Zedong's Selected Works and books by Marx and Lenin. I browsed through them casually. Later, I wandered to the medical section and saw about a dozen books. I picked one up and started flipping through it. Before that, I had never been exposed to such books, and I found them intriguing. So, I bought three books published by the People's Medical Publishing House: "Acupuncture," "Acupuncture Points Chart," and "Textbook for Rural Health Workers." The total cost was a little over 60 cents. I remember it clearly—I took the three books to the cashier and paid for them.

I never imagined that these three books, purchased for just over 60 cents, would determine the path I would follow for the rest of my life...

I am deeply grateful to my late mother. She earned just over 20 yuan a month, yet she had to support both me and my younger sister, and life was tough. Even so, whenever I wanted to buy books, she never hesitated, always saying, "I'll give you the money tomorrow." It wasn't until later that I realized she didn't have any money at the time and had borrowed it from others. My mother often said to our neighbors, "You can save on everything, but you can't skimp on the money for the children to buy books."

Whenever I think of those difficult years when my mother, my sister, and I lived under the weight of political and economic pressures, I feel as though my heart is being torn apart, and tears often stream down my face...

At that time, I was naive enough to think that learning acupuncture was not difficult. I later bought ten needles and started practicing on myself while reading the books.

One day, my mother had a headache, so I tried needling her at acupuncture points such as Taiyang, Baihui, Fengchi, and Hegu. Remarkably, her headache disappeared. Soon, neighbors, their colleagues, friends, classmates, and even their parents began coming to me for acupuncture. Almost every day, someone would show up at my house seeking treatment. This continued for a year and a half, during which I learned while practicing.

Saving lives and healing patients gave me more experience in emergency care.

In December 1968, my classmates and I went to a poor village in Yuanping County, Shanxi Province, to settle as part of the "down to the countryside" movement.

In the first week after settling there, one of my classmates had a stomachache. I performed acupuncture on him at Neiguan, Zhongwan, and Zusanli points, and within a few minutes, his pain subsided. A few days later, an old man in the village also had stomach pain, and after I performed acupuncture on him, his pain disappeared in just a few minutes as well. Soon, word spread throughout the village: "There's a young educated man from Beijing who knows how to treat illnesses."

At that time, I could only handle simple cases like headaches, toothaches, stomachaches, arm pain, back pain, and leg pain, often consulting my books in front of the patients. During the eight years I spent in the countryside, I eagerly studied both traditional Chinese medicine and Western medicine, filling my bookshelves with medical books. I pulled teeth, delivered babies, cleaned and sutured wounds, and treated common conditions in internal medicine, surgery, gynecology, pediatrics, dermatology, and otolaryngology. I also managed to save patients suffering from acute left heart failure, severe asthma, upper gastrointestinal bleeding, various types of shock, and acute organophosphate poisoning. Eventually, people from other counties, even those over a hundred miles away, came to see me. Several local newspapers and radio stations reported on my work treating villagers.

Later on, a delegation from the Beijing Revolutionary Committee came to visit the educated youth in the countryside. After learning about the conditions in our small clinic, they asked me to write a list of the medicines and equipment we needed. I handed them the list, and they allocated over 1,000 yuan for us to purchase supplies. Though 1,000 yuan may seem insignificant today, it was an astronomical sum at the time—I could never have earned that much in 10 years in the village. With that, our small clinic was completely transformed...

Whenever I recall those years in Shanxi, I feel a deep gratitude toward the villagers, who entrusted their lives to me in times of crisis and placed their unwavering trust in me. Though my medical knowledge was limited, they never doubted my skills; though I wasn't a noble person, they never questioned my ethics. Even when a treatment failed, they sincerely thanked me, and that provided immense comfort during those difficult years.

Every time I successfully treated a patient and received praise and gratitude from others, I would always say that it was the simple, honest villagers who nurtured me, enabling me to pursue this noble profession that I love deeply.

Returning Home, Continuing with Emergency Care

After the Cultural Revolution ended, I was fortunate enough to attend university and receive a formal medical education. That too was an unforgettable time.

I remember once during a lecture, the teacher approached me and quietly asked, "Why aren't you taking notes?" I replied, "What you've said that I already know, I didn't take notes on; what you've said that's in the book, I didn't write down either. But what you said that I didn't know and isn't in the book, you can see I've noted it down in the book." The teacher looked and nodded, saying, "Good. That way you can focus better on listening, and it's more effective."

After graduating in 1980, I finally returned to my hometown of Beijing after being away for 12 years. Not long after, I started working at the Beijing Sports Science Research Institute, located in the Beijing Municipal Sports Committee compound near Xiannongtan. There, I conducted research in sports medicine, which was a relatively unfamiliar field for me, and I had to learn a lot of new professional knowledge to adapt to the job. In contrast, clinical medicine was still familiar territory for me, as I had "practiced medicine illegally" for nine and a half years before university, accumulating some clinical experience, so I preferred clinical work. At the time, after returning to Beijing, I didn't know many people. Before joining the Sports Science Research Institute, I approached several hospitals and the municipal and district health bureaus, but they all turned me down because there were no available "quotas." Despite this, I always longed to work in a hospital, where I could treat patients and save lives.

In early 1983, shortly after the Spring Festival, *Beijing Evening News* published an article about the work at the Beijing Emergency Medical Station. I remember one particular sentence from the article: "The personnel and equipment at the Beijing Emergency Medical Station are far from meeting the needs of the capital city's political status and the practical needs of its people." After reading this article, especially that sentence, I felt my blood boil with excitement. Without much thought, that evening, I wrote a letter to the leadership of the Beijing Emergency Medical Station, expressing my passion for emergency care and my desire to work at the station. Later, the station's director told me that he was so impressed with my letter that he read it to the entire medical staff. To my surprise, on the afternoon of the third day after sending the letter, the station's director, the renowned emergency care expert Professor Li Zonghao, arranged an interview with me. Right there and then, he decided to offer me a job at the emergency station.

However, the leadership at the Sports Science Research Institute didn't want me to leave. Back then, wanting to switch jobs was considered a sign of "not being content with one's current job," and it often resulted in the person being unable to move, leaving a bad impression on others. It wasn't like today, where people can change jobs, even frequently, without much issue. My highly respected institute director spoke to me earnestly, saying, "You are simple-minded and straightforward, and so are our colleagues here. This place is very suitable for you. There aren't many units like ours. If you go to a place with complex personnel relationships, I'm afraid you won't be able to adapt. Besides, we also need you here, so we really don't want you to leave."

I indeed felt very reluctant to part with my colleagues at the institute. They were all simple, kind, warm-hearted, intelligent, and resilient. Most of them were former top athletes, including some award-winning athletes and renowned coaches, as well as university graduates from prestigious institutions before the Cultural Revolution. To this day, I often feel guilty for not living up to the director's expectations and for leaving despite his kindness. But for the sake of my passion for emergency care, I persisted in this path until retirement—a journey that lasted nearly 30 years.

Joining the Beijing Emergency Medical Center

In October 1949, the People's Republic of China was founded. However, Beijing was already liberated in February of that year, and various government institutions, including the Beijing Health Bureau, were established shortly after. At the time, Beijing had only one captured American Jeep, which had been painted with a bright red cross and equipped with a large, shiny bronze bell. The bell was about 40 centimeters tall and looked quite heavy. It was hung on the right side of the ambulance, and the doctor would shake it, producing a loud, pleasant sound that could be heard from far away. When I was a child, I saw this ambulance speeding down the street and heard the sound of that bell. Later, when I started working at the emergency station, I also saw the big bell. I'm not sure where it ended up now, but I'm certain that many older Beijingers around my age or older would remember it.

In the past, the working and living conditions at the Beijing Emergency Medical Station were extremely poor, incomparable to the Beijing Emergency Medical Center today. We only had a rickety ambulance that rattled loudly when it moved, a single medical kit, an oxygen bag, a driver, and a doctor. That was the entirety of our resources when responding to emergencies. In many cases, this equipment was far from sufficient. At the time, the entire emergency station had only two electrocardiograph machines, both made in Shanghai, powered by multiple D-sized batteries, and weighing more than 5 kilograms. We also had one defibrillator, which was so heavy that it took two people to carry it. To make matters worse, the electrocardiograph machine was sometimes taken by other doctors, leaving us without one when attending to heart attack patients. All we could rely on was our experience and verbal communication to assess the situation.

As the saying goes, "To do a good job, one must first sharpen one's tools." I realized that the current situation couldn't continue. So I approached our department head, Fu Daqing, and shared my thoughts: we needed a fully equipped rescue vehicle for critical emergencies. A few days later, Fu Daqing asked me to write a list of the emergency equipment required for such a vehicle. Soon after, four modern emergency vehicles, fully equipped with advanced medical devices, arrived at our station. These vehicles were equipped with imported electrocardiographs, defibrillator monitors, ventilators, suction machines, endotracheal tubes, and other portable equipment, all compact and lightweight, perfect for use in the field.

While this may not seem extraordinary today, at the time, it was a groundbreaking achievement for the Beijing Emergency Medical Station. From that moment on, I spent over 20 years accompanying these advanced rescue vehicles, working in emergency care until my retirement.

Today, the ambulances of the Beijing Emergency Medical Center are even more advanced, equipped with devices like electric chest compression pumps and electronic video laryngoscopes, making emergency care more efficient and convenient.

In 1955, the Beijing Emergency Medical Station was officially established. Officially, Beijing's pre-hospital emergency care is generally considered to have begun in 1955, but I believe it actually started in 1949.

Old Beijingers will remember that the Beijing Emergency Medical Station was located on Nan Chi Zi Street, next to Tiananmen Square, and the emergency phone number at the time was 5678 in the fifth telephone district. This number originally belonged to the sister of Mr. Le Songsheng, the deputy mayor of Beijing and the owner of the Tongrentang Pharmacy. To make it easier for citizens to remember, they gave this number to the emergency station. Later, with telephone upgrades, the number was changed to 55-5678 and 6525-5678. In 1988, when the Beijing Emergency Medical Center was officially established, the nationwide emergency number 120 was introduced, but 6525-5678 is still in use today. If 120 is unavailable, you can still call 6525-5678.

During the decades I spent in emergency care, there were moments of joy and sorrow, but what sustained me was my unwavering commitment and passion for the work. I am grateful to my mother, to the kind-hearted villagers who supported me, and to my colleagues, friends, and loved ones who have always stood by me. Although I am now retired, I continue to dedicate myself to advancing emergency care in China, helping more people learn first aid and self-rescue skills, so they can do more than just call 120 when faced with an accident or injury.

Pre-Hospital Emergency Success Rates Reflect a Society's Level of Civilization

Many people believe that doctors, especially emergency physicians, are cold and indifferent. They think that since we face death daily, we must have become numb and apathetic toward life. I've been asked many times: "Since you're dealing with life and death every day, have you become desensitized to human life?"

My response is always the same: "In fact, quite the opposite. Precisely because we deal with life and death daily, we have a deeper and more profound appreciation for life and a greater respect for the dignity of life. We aren't indifferent to life. It's just that we've experienced so much that our psychological resilience is much stronger than that of the average person."

The word "emergency" has two components: "urgent," meaning every second counts, and "rescue," meaning doing everything possible to save a life. Emergency care is a battle with death, a fight to pull people back from the brink of the underworld. Sudden cardiac arrest is the gateway to that underworld. Those who survive after being rescued have essentially taken a round trip to see the King of Hell and returned. Those who are not saved remain there forever.

Modern emergency care mainly consists of three

parts: pre-hospital emergency care, continued treatment in the emergency department, and more specialized care in critical care units (like the ICU, CCU, etc.).

Pre-hospital emergency care, also called out-of-hospital or on-site emergency care, refers to assistance provided outside of hospitals, at any time or place, before the patient enters a hospital. It focuses on acute, life-threatening conditions and emergencies, ensuring that patients are swiftly and safely removed from dangerous environments. It involves rapid assessment, rescue, care, transport, and continuous monitoring en route to the hospital, buying time for life-saving interventions and further hospital care.

In its narrow definition, pre-hospital emergency care is handled by emergency centers. Broadly speaking, it should include not only emergency centers and hospitals but also community health service centers (clinics), outpatient departments, infirmaries, and health stations. It should also include universal self-help and mutual assistance. Pre-hospital emergency care is an irreplaceable component of modern emergency medicine, serving as the front line in medical rescue efforts and often the last line of defense in saving lives.

What constitutes an acute and critical condition? For instance, if someone suddenly has a fever, is that an emergency? Yes, it's urgent but not critical, and it's not life-threatening. The patient can usually go to the emergency room on their own or with help from family. On the other hand, a liver cancer patient is critically ill, but it's not urgent. They may not need an ambulance or even emergency care; they can receive treatment or be admitted to the hospital through outpatient services.

There are many types of acute illnesses—some occur suddenly, while others are exacerbations of chronic conditions. Some can quickly become life-threatening, while others may lead to life-threatening situations if not treated promptly. Some conditions, though not life-threatening, cause great suffering for the patient. Others may not be life-threatening, nor cause significant discomfort for the patient... Therefore, the severity of various acute illnesses differs.

So, when do you need an emergency physician? If a feverish patient suddenly starts convulsing or loses consciousness, or if a liver cancer patient experiences massive bleeding due to ruptured esophageal or gastric varices, both patients are critically ill and at risk of death. In such cases, you must immediately call emergency number 120, and that's when we emergency doctors step in!

Who should you rely on when a sudden cardiac arrest occurs and someone's life is at stake? In my opinion, you cannot solely rely on doctors or emergency centers.

Why do I say this? From the time of the onset of the condition to the moment someone thinks to dial the emergency number, the phone call is made, the situation is explained, and the address is clarified, followed by the dispatching of doctors and vehicles by the emergency center, and the ambulance racing to the patient's location—all of these steps take time. If everything goes smoothly, the doctor may arrive in under 15 minutes. However, if things go wrong—such as the emergency line being busy, or the hospital being understaffed, or encountering traffic jams—the situation becomes less optimistic.

Countless times, we've rushed to the scene only to be met with disgruntled family members: "What took you so long? Why are you so late?" In those moments, no matter how wronged we feel, we have to endure it and understand that the family is anxious.

In the United States, an average of 450,000 people experience sudden cardiac arrest each year. As early as the 1980s, the survival rate in Seattle was as high as 43%. In contrast, China experiences about 544,000 sudden cardiac deaths annually, but the survival rate is less than 1%. Why is there such a vast gap between China and the U.S. in terms of resuscitation success rates?

I have data from 2008: In Seattle, emergency response time was under 5 minutes, with a response radius of 2 to 3 kilometers and one ambulance per 20,000 to 30,000 people. Emergency preparedness reached 70% of the population. In Beijing, however, the average emergency response time was 15 minutes, with a response radius of 5 to 7 kilometers and one ambulance per 100,000 people. During the busiest times, the Beijing Emergency Medical Center could receive over 20,000 emergency calls and dispatch more than 2,000 vehicles in a day, but even that was not enough to meet the demand. During the Olympics, Beijing aimed to have one in every 80 residents trained in emergency care, but even then, the rate of emergency preparedness was far below that of Western countries.

Many times, we've arrived at the scene as quickly as possible, only to find the patient already dead, with those around them standing by helplessly, not knowing how to provide first aid. This makes it clear that the Chinese public lacks not only emergency knowledge, skills, and equipment but also emergency awareness.

The level of emergency preparedness and the success rate of resuscitation, including CPR, is not just an indicator of a country's medical development but also a measure of its economic prosperity, urban management, social cohesion, the government's attention to public welfare, and the overall quality of its citizens. It has become a key marker of the civilization and harmony of a nation, a city, or an organization.

The government and society should incorporate internationally-minded health education, emergency care training, and death education into lifelong compulsory education for all. Especially in high-risk and service industries, emergency skills should be a required professional competency. In schools at all levels, emergency care training should be a compulsory subject!

In cases of sudden cardiac arrest, the most crucial factor is immediate first aid by those nearby. It's essential to act promptly, accurately, and persistently! Don't assume that calling an ambulance is enough. Before the emergency doctor arrives, initiating on-site self-rescue and mutual assistance is the only way to save lives—and that's the true significance of learning first aid.

Chapter 1: Sudden Death: Pulling People Back from the Brink of Death

The "Chief of Demons": A Mighty Opponent

Emergency at the Scene

As the saying goes, "The sky can change unexpectedly, and so can fortune." Many people believe that only middle-aged and elderly individuals are at risk of sudden death, but this is far from the truth. In fact, cases of sudden death among young people are becoming increasingly common.

The first time I handled an emergency rescue mission on my own was shortly after I started working at the Beijing Emergency Medical Center, and it involved rescuing a young man. At that time, sudden death among young people was rare—he was only in his thirties. That experience left a deep impression on me.

It was early morning in late June, just as dawn was breaking, when I received the dispatch to head out. There were very few people or cars on the streets at the time, unlike today when the traffic at night surpasses the amount from the daytime back then. Our ambulance quickly reached the entrance of an alley where a person who had called for the ambulance got in and guided us, saying, "It doesn't look good—he's already not breathing."

From the introduction, I learned what had happened: that morning, around 5 a.m., the wife woke up to use the bathroom and found that her husband wasn't in bed. When she went to the outer room, she saw him lying on the floor, unresponsive no matter how much she called him. In panic, she ran into the courtyard and yelled for the neighbors. Several neighbors, startled awake from their sleep, rushed out to see what was happening. Some of them quickly realized the severity of the situation and called the emergency hotline.

Carrying our rescue equipment, we quickly got out of the ambulance and ran into the courtyard. Upon entering the house, we saw a man in his thirties lying on the floor of the outer room. His wife stood beside him, and next to her was a little boy, about three or four years old, squatting by his side, seemingly too young to understand what had happened. A crowd of neighbors stood around both inside and outside, watching, but no one attempted to rescue him.

I rushed forward and squatted down to examine the patient. He was already unconscious, with cyanosis on his face and lips. There was no breathing, pulse, or heartbeat. His body was cold, and dark red livor mortis had already appeared on the parts of his body that were pressed against the floor. His limbs were stiff, and all his joints had lost flexibility. It was clear that rigor mortis had set in, and with the appearance of coldness, lividity, and stiffness, it was already too late to save him.

I stood up and told the family, "The patient has died, his body is stiff, and he's been dead for at least one or two hours. There's no way to save him."

As soon as I finished speaking, the wife burst into tears. The little boy, not understanding what had happened, clung to his mother's leg, frightened by her sudden outburst of sobbing.

Crying himself, he kept repeating, "Mommy, don't cry. Mommy, don't cry..." The boy was trying to comfort his mother while crying himself.

Some neighbors pleaded with me, "Doctor, please try to save him. Maybe there's still hope for a miracle." Others commented, "What's the point of saving him? He's already stiff—it's too late."

After the initial commotion had settled down, I explained to everyone, "This young man died of sudden cardiac death. Although sudden death is dangerous, it's not always impossible to bring someone back to life."

Their eyes lit up with a glimmer of hope.

I continued, "If a person's heart stops and breathing ceases for no more than 4 to 6 minutes, there's a good chance they can be revived. However, once more time passes, the brain suffers permanent damage. If it's been more than 10 minutes, the person becomes brain-dead, and it's virtually impossible to revive them. If we act within that 4 to 6-minute window and provide prompt first aid, we might be able to save the patient. So, those 4 to 6 minutes are crucial. However, in this case, the patient has already shown signs of rigor mortis. Rigor mortis and livor mortis usually appear 2 to 4 hours after death, depending on the environment and temperature—sooner in winter, later in summer. This means the patient has been dead for at least two hours, and at this point, it's impossible to revive him. If someone had known how to perform CPR and had acted immediately upon discovering the patient, this young man might have had a chance to survive!"

The neighbors fell silent, some nodding in agreement. After that, they started explaining more about the young man's life. I learned that he was outwardly strong and healthy, with a robust appetite and a love for smoking and drinking. He was also known for his great strength and bad temper. His snoring at night was so loud that even the neighbors could hear it from the courtyard.

I asked, "Did he have any health problems?"

Everyone responded in unison, "No, he was always in great shape."

However, I also learned that both of his parents had a history of high blood pressure, coronary heart disease, and diabetes. His mother had suffered a stroke a few years ago and was still unable to take care of herself. His father had been hospitalized at Fuwai Hospital the previous year for acute myocardial infarction and had nearly died.

Based on the information provided, I suspected that the young man had likely died of sudden cardiac death due to his family's history of cardiovascular disease. Even if he appeared healthy on the outside, individuals in such families need to be particularly vigilant about cardiovascular disease and the risk of sudden death.

By the time we returned to the emergency center that day, the sun was already high in the sky. The driver was sweating profusely, but I felt cold to my core, both physically and mentally. I felt particularly miserable. Even though the young man's death had nothing to do with me, I couldn't help but feel shaken—he was in his thirties, just like me at the time, and his death reminded me of life's fragility.

I couldn't stop thinking about his home. Although the furnishings were simple, everything was neat and clean, radiating a sense of warmth. It was clearly a happy little family. But this sudden disaster had left behind a widow and an orphan, breaking my heart...

Now, that little boy would be around 40 years old. He's probably married with children by now, and his own child might even be in elementary school. His mother would be in her sixties. Although I've long forgotten what the mother and son looked like, I can still vividly remember what happened that morning.

Over my 30 years in emergency medicine, I've witnessed cases of sudden death every day. Many of the victims have been young people in their twenties and thirties. In recent years, the number of sudden deaths among young people has significantly increased due to work pressure. There are far more cases now than when I first joined the Beijing Emergency Medical Center, and incidents of sudden death among middle-aged and elderly people have become even more common.

So, what exactly is sudden death?

Sudden death, as the term suggests, refers to unexpected, rapid death. It occurs when a seemingly healthy person or someone whose condition is stable dies suddenly, unexpectedly, and naturally within 6 hours of the onset of symptoms. Of these, cardiac-related sudden deaths account for over 80%, and whether or not the patient has a history of heart disease, death typically occurs within 1 hour of onset.

The definition of "within 6 hours" is consistent with regulations in China and the World Health Organization (WHO). In some countries or regions, the time limit is extended to 12 or 24 hours. While these time frames are not absolute, they serve as general guidelines.

The renowned comedian Hou Yaowen passed away more than 6 hours after he first started experiencing symptoms. He began feeling back pain in the morning and died around 6 p.m. Despite exceeding the 6-hour limit (let alone 1 hour), his death was still classified as sudden cardiac death, and this diagnosis is widely accepted in the medical field.

The three defining characteristics of sudden death are its suddenness, unexpectedness, and natural cause.

"Sudden" refers to the rapid onset, and "unexpected" means it was unforeseen. These terms are self-explanatory, understood by even young children. However, the concept of "natural" death is not as widely understood.

A "natural" death occurs as a result of disease, following the natural course of illness without any external or violent intervention. It does not include "unnatural deaths" or violent deaths caused by factors other than disease, such as electrocution, drowning, suicide, acute poisoning, car accidents, falls, workplace accidents, or homicide.

Among all diseases, in terms of suddenness, urgency, danger, and consequences, nothing compares to sudden death. For this reason, sudden death has earned the title of the "chief of demons."

Clinically, sudden death is divided into two major categories: cardiac and non-cardiac sudden death.

Cardiac sudden death, also known as heart-related sudden death, occurs when the heart is the primary cause of the patient's sudden death. Whether or not the patient has a history of heart disease, death occurs within an hour of onset. This is the most common type of sudden death.

Generally, cardiac sudden death is caused by two main types of heart disease. One is coronary artery disease, with acute myocardial infarction being the most severe form and the leading cause of sudden death, accounting for 80% to 90% of all sudden deaths. The other type includes non-coronary heart diseases, such as myocarditis, cardiomyopathy, heart valve disease, aortic dissection aneurysm, congenital and acquired QT syndrome, and Brugada syndrome.

Non-cardiac sudden death, also known as non-heart-related sudden death, refers to sudden death caused by factors unrelated to the heart. This type accounts for 10% to 20% of all sudden deaths.

I often say, "Sudden death is an extreme challenge to both humanity and medicine." The reason I say this is that the defining characteristics of emergency tasks are their sudden onset and time sensitivity, and among them, sudden death is the most urgent, the most critical, and the most dangerous. The golden window to save a life is often just a few minutes. This requires emergency personnel to arrive at the scene promptly, make quick and accurate assessments, and provide immediate treatment. If there's one situation that best exemplifies "every second counts," it's the rescue of a patient experiencing sudden death. This perfectly embodies the emergency medicine principle that "time is life."

Sudden Yet Not Unexpected: The Signs of Sudden Death

Emergency Scene

Although sudden death seems to strike out of nowhere, catching people off guard, if you observe carefully, you'll find that some patients actually show warning signs before it happens. Unfortunately, many people fail to recognize and take these critical signals seriously.

This reminds me of the time I tried to save Vice Mayor Li Runwu of Beijing.

On November 2, 1995, the Beijing Municipal Government was scheduled to hold a meeting at 9 a.m. that day. By then, all the attendees from various bureaus and offices had already arrived, and the meeting was about to start. Mayor Li Qiyan, Executive Vice Mayor Zhang Baifa, and Vice Mayor Li Runwu had a brief conversation in a small meeting room adjacent to the main conference hall. Then, Mayor Li Qiyan stood up and said, "Let's go." Vice Mayor Zhang Baifa stood up as well, but they both noticed that Vice Mayor Li Runwu was still sitting on the sofa, motionless and unresponsive. They called out to him loudly, "Runwu, Runwu!" The clock showed it was 8:58 a.m.

Mayor Li Qiyan quickly pushed the door open and shouted to the people waiting outside, "Does anyone have heart medication?" A leader from the Municipal Procuratorate hurriedly took out some nitroglycerin and handed it to the mayor, who personally placed the pill in Vice Mayor Li Runwu's mouth. Meanwhile, Vice Mayor Zhang Baifa instructed the staff to call both the government medical office and the emergency center.

I was ordered to rush to the city government to save the vice mayor. The ambulance arrived at 9:10 a.m., and the incident had taken place in a small meeting room inside the city government, where the hallways were already crowded with people. As soon as we arrived, they cleared a path for us, and we quickly ran to the patient's side. The head of the government medical office, Director Jiang, was kneeling on the floor, performing chest compressions. The patient had no heartbeat or breathing, so the nurse and I immediately administered medication, intubated the patient, and connected the heart monitor, which displayed a flat line. We did everything we could to save him while Vice Mayor Zhang Baifa explained the situation.

After several rounds of chest compressions, artificial respiration, and correcting acidosis, the patient's electrocardiogram showed ventricular fibrillation a few times, and each time we promptly defibrillated him, but it would immediately revert to a flat line. After another 10 minutes, Vice Mayor He Luli, who was a doctor herself, arrived at the scene, followed by Professor Li Zonghao, the deputy director of the Beijing Emergency Center and a renowned emergency expert. Specialists from Beijing Hospital and Beijing Tongren Hospital also came to help. Despite the collective efforts of all these top experts, the patient showed no response. Vice Mayor Zhang Baifa quietly said to me, "At 10 o'clock, I could tell there was no hope." I replied, "Didn't I say from the moment I arrived that there was a 100% chance of no success but a 100% effort?" In fact, all the doctors, nurses, and most people present already understood the situation—they just didn't want to say it out loud.

In the end, the experts and leaders decided to transfer the patient to the nearby Beijing Tongren Hospital for further rescue efforts. The doctors exchanged knowing glances, fully aware of what this meant. By then, it was already past 11 a.m. As expected, the final outcome was inevitable: 56-year-old Vice Mayor Li Runwu had passed away.

In fact, there had been warning signs leading up to Vice Mayor Li's sudden death. His staff mentioned that in the days before his passing, he had been feeling unwell, experiencing fatigue, chest tightness, shortness of breath, and palpitations. Once, on his way to a meeting, he asked the driver to stop the car so he could inhale some oxygen, and after feeling better, he continued on his way. On another occasion, during a meeting, Vice Mayor Li suddenly lost consciousness and slumped under the table. Everyone had urged him to go to the hospital for a checkup, but he always responded, "I'll go after we solve Beijing's winter heating issues." Sadly, he never got the chance to go, leaving this world before that day arrived. This is a reminder that when you suddenly feel unwell or experience unusual symptoms, you should immediately go to the hospital and not take it lightly.

Some patients show no warning signs before sudden death, making it impossible to prevent. In Vice Mayor Li's case, however, there were clear signs, but they weren't taken seriously, and he ultimately couldn't escape his fate. When I was trying to save him, I overheard several staff members saying, "He worked himself to death." Just as sharpening a knife won't delay chopping firewood, seeking timely medical attention when you're ill could help prevent or reduce the chances of a sudden death tragedy.

In reality, most emergencies that cause sudden death have fairly typical symptoms or clear warning signs, but some of these signals are easily overlooked or misdiagnosed. If any of the following symptoms occur, those around the patient should perform whatever first aid they can while immediately calling the emergency number, 120.

Learning Brings Me Joy

Below are symptoms that may indicate the possibility of sudden death:

Atypical Presentations of Death	Diseases That May Accompany
Chest Pain	Acute myocardial infarction, the most dangerous and common condition.
Breathing Difficulty	Acute heart failure, severe dyspnea, shortness of breath, etc.
Palpitations	Ventricular tachycardia, ventricular fibrillation, severe atrial fibrillation causing blockages.
Severe Headache	Acute stroke.

Atypical Presentations of Death	Diseases That May Accompany
Limb Paralysis	Acute stroke and other serious diseases of the nervous system.
Dizziness	Caused by various heart conditions, acute stroke, head trauma, low blood pressure, and other severe conditions.
Convulsions	Could be caused by epilepsy, seizures, febrile convulsions, tetanus, or poisoning by toxins.
Acute Abdominal Pain	Acute pancreatitis, gastrointestinal perforation, acute appendicitis, intestinal obstruction, ectopic pregnancy rupture, abdominal aortic aneurysm rupture, or myocardial infarction presenting as abdominal pain.
Choking	Airway obstruction by foreign objects, vomiting, water, food, etc.

■Chest Pain

Chest pain is not only a symptom of heart disease; many other diseases can also present as chest pain. The most dangerous and common situation for chest pain is acute myocardial infarction. Whenever someone experiences chest pain, people usually think of heart disease first, which helps avoid overlooking this potential danger. However, if heart disease presents with atypical symptoms, it often does not draw enough attention, and acute myocardial infarction may be ignored, leading to sudden death.

I will give a detailed introduction to the typical and atypical manifestations of acute myocardial infarction in the next chapter.

■Breathing Difficulty

Sudden onset of breathing difficulty is often very dangerous. Conditions such as acute left heart failure, severe asthma, and pneumothorax can lead to breathing difficulties, which can quickly become life-threatening.

■Palpitations

Sudden onset of a rapid heart rate, especially exceeding 140 beats per minute, may indicate supraventricular tachycardia. If a supraventricular tachycardia episode lasts a bit longer, it can cause dizziness, fainting, chest pain, low blood pressure, and even shock. If during an acute myocardial infarction, the heart rate suddenly exceeds 100 beats per minute, it may indicate a more dangerous ventricular tachycardia, which is a sign of possible sudden death. If the heart rate suddenly drops below 60 beats per minute, especially below 50 beats per minute, it may indicate severe atrioventricular block, especially if the heart rate slows during acute myocardial infarction, which is also a dangerous signal for sudden death.

■Severe Headache

Patients with a history of high blood pressure who suddenly experience severe headaches accompanied by vomiting may be about to have, or are already experiencing, acute cerebrovascular disease, which can easily lead to sudden death.

■Limb Paralysis

This could involve paralysis of one side of the body, one limb, both legs, or all four limbs, indicating the occurrence of acute cerebrovascular disease or other serious conditions of the nervous system, and is also a dangerous signal for sudden death.

■Coma

A patient who suddenly falls into a coma, meaning they cannot be awakened no matter how much you call them, could be experiencing cardiac arrest, acute cerebrovascular disease, head trauma, hypoglycemia, various acute poisonings, or other critical conditions.

■Convulsions

Convulsions may be caused by a major seizure of epilepsy, hysteria, high fever in children, or could occur at the moment of cardiac arrest. Many elderly people with heart disease spend a long time doing one thing, such as playing mahjong, combined with stuffy, poorly ventilated weather, which can easily lead to convulsions, heavy sweating, pale face, and sudden death. In some cases, young people without regular exercise habits suddenly engage in intense physical activity, leading to convulsions and sudden death.

■Acute Abdominal Pain

Acute pancreatitis, gastrointestinal perforation, acute appendicitis, acute cholecystitis, intestinal obstruction, and ectopic pregnancy rupture can all cause abdominal pain. Upper abdominal pain can also be a symptom of acute myocardial infarction. Acute hemorrhagic necrotizing pancreatitis, ectopic pregnancy rupture, and acute myocardial infarction can rapidly become life-threatening. In addition, conditions like aortic dissection and severe pulmonary embolism, where patients may experience cardiac arrest, can also present with abdominal pain.

■Choking

Choking can occur due to airway obstruction from foreign bodies, laryngeal edema, or injuries to the face and neck, leading to a lack of oxygen as the lungs cannot exchange gases with the outside environment. The patient may have severe coughing, difficulty breathing, cyanosis or pale complexion, restlessness, consciousness disorders, and respiratory or cardiac arrest.

■Other Situations

Sudden, severe increases in blood pressure can lead to acute cerebrovascular disease or acute left heart failure. If blood pressure suddenly drops sharply, shock should be considered. Vomiting blood can occur with gastrointestinal ulcers, liver cirrhosis, or esophageal varices rupture. Hemoptysis (coughing up blood) may be seen in tuberculosis, and these situations can lead to shock or suffocation due to bleeding, threatening life. Sudden dizziness or vertigo (feeling of the surroundings spinning or the person spinning) can be a sign of acute cerebrovascular disease. There are also situations like acute poisoning, electric shock, drowning, hanging, and other sudden, serious, and painful emergencies.

Statistics show that approximately 90% of all sudden death cases occur outside of hospitals in various settings, with only a small percentage happening inside hospitals.
Of these, 65% of people die within 15 minutes of

the onset of symptoms, often before they have time to go to the hospital, and it is unlikely that an ambulance will reach them within 4 minutes. As a result, they die in various locations outside the hospital.

The remaining 35% die between 15 minutes and 2 hours after the onset of symptoms. Obviously, some patients also don't make it to the hospital and die at the scene of the onset or on the way to the hospital. Why is it that two hours is still not enough time, and why do some still die outside the hospital? This is often because their symptoms were atypical and did not draw enough attention from the patient or their family. For example, Mr. Hou Yaowen did not experience chest pain but back pain at the time, and it wasn't taken seriously enough, which led to his sudden death.

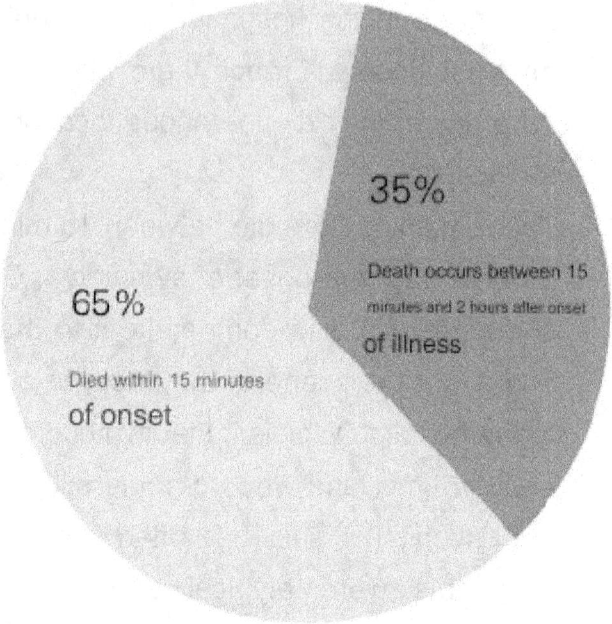

35%
Death occurs between 15
minutes and 2 hours after onset
of illness

65%
Died within 15 minutes
of onset

Are You at High Risk of Sudden Death?

Someone once asked me: "Dr. Jia, can you predict whether I will die suddenly? When will it happen?" Every time, I firmly respond: "No! I am not a deity, I cannot predict that. But I can assess whether someone belongs to a high-risk group for sudden death."

If a person belongs to a high-risk group, their chances of experiencing sudden death naturally increase. So, who are considered high-risk for sudden death?

Middle-aged and Elderly People Aged 50-70

As life expectancy increases and our society ages, our country will gradually align with developed countries and face the peak incidence of coronary heart disease. Overall, the incidence rate is higher in middle-aged and elderly people compared to younger individuals, and higher in young people compared to minors.

Incidence of Sudden Death:

■ People with a Family History of Chronic Diseases

In families where parents have chronic diseases such as arteriosclerosis, hypertension, coronary heart disease, cerebrovascular disease, or diabetes, the likelihood of children developing these diseases is higher. Conversely, if parents do not have these diseases, their children have a lower chance of developing them.

Although coronary heart disease is not hereditary, it does tend to run in families. Other risk factors for coronary heart disease, such as hypertension, hyperlipidemia, diabetes, and obesity, also play a role.

Additionally, family members often share similar or even identical lifestyle habits, and sometimes even similar personalities and behavior due to long-term cohabitation, which can become risk factors.

The United States was once one of the countries with a high incidence of coronary heart disease. If we were to follow the general concept of inheritance or family history, there would certainly be many more "coronary heart disease families" in the U.S. than in China, and their offspring's incidence rates would also increase. However, in recent years, the incidence of coronary heart disease in the U.S. has dropped significantly, which is closely related to the country's growing advocacy for a healthy lifestyle.

■ People with Type A Personality

People with Type A personalities are stubborn, impatient, meticulous, and often have tense relationships, with a constant sense of urgency. Type A personalities can be divided into two types:

- The first type speaks quickly, walks fast, is stubborn, impatient, competitive, decisive, impulsive, and prone to bursts of anger. These individuals tend to have higher levels of adrenaline in their blood and are more prone to developing hypertension, coronary heart disease, etc.

- The second type is more introverted but still impatient and easily excited. However, they tend to suppress their emotions, and even if they are dissatisfied, they do not show it. They often experience suppressed anger and frustration. This second type tends to have even higher levels of adrenaline than the first and is more prone to hypertension, coronary heart disease, etc., with their conditions progressing faster.

Every time I encounter a patient with acute myocardial infarction, cerebral hemorrhage, or sudden death, I often ask their family members: "How was their temper?" The response is often, "Their temper was not good," "They had a really bad temper," or "They were very irritable."
People with Type A personalities generally have higher cholesterol levels in their blood vessels, shorter clotting times, and slower blood flow of red blood cells. Type A personalities are not only a risk factor for arteriosclerosis but can also directly trigger sudden onset of serious conditions such as angina, acute myocardial infarction, blood pressure spikes, cerebral hemorrhage, or sudden death due to emotional outbursts. Therefore, learning to control emotions is crucial to preventing tragedy.

■ Patients with Latent Coronary Heart Disease

Some people "appear healthy" but may actually have underlying or undiagnosed diseases such as heart disease. We encounter such patients almost every day, especially relatively younger individuals in their 40s, 50s, or even 20s and 30s.

When we arrive at the scene, the patient's heart and breathing have often already stopped. While rescuing them, we ask those around about the patient's medical history: "What happened just before?" If there are people around, they can usually explain clearly. We continue to ask, "What illnesses did they have in the past?" Often, we hear answers like, "They never had any illnesses; they were in great shape."

But can someone with no illness really die? Can someone who was "in great shape" really die? Such statements are inaccurate. It's not that they had no illness; rather, it's that "they were unaware of any illnesses," "nothing had been discovered," or "they had never been diagnosed." These statements are more objective. Of course, as doctors, we can't expect people to always phrase it this way.

There is a subtype of coronary heart disease called "asymptomatic myocardial ischemia," also known as "latent coronary heart disease" or "asymptomatic coronary heart disease." As the name implies, the patient has coronary heart disease but without symptoms. Since they don't feel anything, they believe they don't have heart disease, but in reality, they do. They just don't know it, and others believe they are healthy.

A U.S. statistic shows that among all coronary heart disease patients, 25% of them present with sudden death as their first symptom. The most common first symptoms of coronary heart disease are chest tightness and shortness of breath, though some patients experience chest pain, palpitations, breathing difficulty, loss of consciousness, or shock during their first episode. The most common symptoms are still chest tightness and shortness of breath, but 25% of patients experience sudden death without ever having shown these symptoms.

■ Postmenopausal Women

In general, the rate of sudden death in men is much higher than in women. Some statistics suggest that the ratio of sudden death in men to women is as high as 4:1 or even 7:1. This may be related to men bearing more family and societal pressures, as well as unhealthy habits such as smoking, excessive drinking, and staying up late. Therefore, men should pay more attention to adopting a healthy lifestyle to stay further away from sudden death.

It is worth noting that the incidence rate in premenopausal women is lower than that of men, but postmenopausal women see a gradual increase in incidence, approaching the levels seen in men. This is related to changes in hormone levels. Of course, women should also adopt a healthy lifestyle, or they risk facing the same danger. Women in their 20s can also experience sudden death, and for postmenopausal women, the risk is even higher if they do not take precautions.

■ People in Certain Professions

Sudden death is more common among people in unhealthy lifestyles, irregular work schedules, overworked conditions, and those under high psychological pressure. High-risk groups include intellectuals, white-collar workers, entertainers, athletes, entrepreneurs, police officers, taxi drivers, government employees, and others.

While the people mentioned above are at high risk for sudden death, being in a high-risk group does not guarantee that sudden death will occur. As the saying goes, "Preparation leads to success; lack of preparation leads to failure." Staying away from sudden death not only requires being aware of risk factors but also involves adjusting one's lifestyle. Additionally, people in high-risk groups should especially be equipped with some basic first-aid knowledge.

"Learning Brings Me Joy"

Beware of the Following High-Risk Factors for Sudden Death

Factors	Description
Age Factors	Middle-aged and elderly people aged 50–70 years are most at risk, followed by those aged 40–50 years. People under 40 and over 70

Factors	Description
	years have a lower risk.
Genetic Factors	A family history of atherosclerosis, hypertension, coronary heart disease, cerebrovascular disease, diabetes, and other chronic diseases increases the likelihood of these conditions in children.
Personality Factors	Individuals with Type A blood tend to have higher levels of renal enzymes in their blood, making them more susceptible to hypertension, coronary heart disease, and related conditions.
Other Factors	Gender-wise, men are more at risk than women, while post-menopausal women have a higher risk than men of the same age. Occupations involving high stress levels can increase the risk of death. People with a history of cancer are more likely to die, such as those with a "hidden health condition" related to heart disease or latent coronary heart disease.

Avoid the "Four Major Danger Zones" and Never Become a Victim

The causes of sudden death are mostly related to unhealthy lifestyles, which also contribute to many chronic diseases. These factors greatly expand the potential for sudden death.

■ Smoking

Smoking offers no benefits and is one of the most significant risk factors for coronary heart disease. It is also the easiest risk factor to avoid and the only one that harms both the smoker and others.

Smoking not only causes respiratory diseases such as lung cancer and pulmonary heart disease, but it also has a more severe impact on the cardiovascular system. It can cause coronary artery spasms and increased heart rate, leading to myocardial ischemia. More dangerously, smoking directly damages the endothelial cells of blood vessels, stripping them of protection, causing lipid accumulation on the vessel walls, and promoting the formation of atherosclerosis. Damage to the vascular intima can also cause platelets to adhere and aggregate, leading to thrombosis, which may result in acute myocardial infarction, cerebral infarction, and more. The longer and heavier the smoking habit, the higher the incidence of hypertension, coronary heart disease, cerebrovascular disease, etc. Smokers are 2 to 10 times more likely to develop coronary heart disease compared to non-smokers.

My longtime friend, brother, and mentor, Professor Hu Dayi, a renowned expert in cardiovascular disease, pointed out in his article *Tobacco Control Is Key to Reducing Premature Deaths from Chronic Diseases* that "globally, tobacco-related deaths account for 10% of cardiovascular deaths. Notably, in people under 45, more than one-third (35%) of cardiovascular deaths are attributed to smoking. Among the risk factors for myocardial infarction in young people, smoking has the greatest impact. Tobacco is the leading risk factor for myocardial infarction, cardiovascular death, and the increasing occurrence of sudden death among younger people. In China, secondhand smoke significantly increases the risk of cardiovascular disease among non-smokers, especially women. Simply reducing secondhand smoke exposure in public places can lead to a marked decrease (30%-40%) in the incidence of acute myocardial infarction within a year."

Professor Hu also emphasized, "Smoking, including secondhand smoke, is a risk factor for all chronic diseases. Effective tobacco control benefits the management of all chronic diseases. Without genuine tobacco control, the dream of a healthy China cannot be realized."

Other risk factors mostly harm only the individual, but smoking not only harms the smoker but also others. Rejecting secondhand smoke is an effective way to reduce smoking rates.

■ Unhealthy Diet

This includes high-fat, high-salt, and high-sugar diets, along with frequent excessive drinking. These dietary patterns are unreasonable and promote the formation of atherosclerosis, which is a major risk factor for hypertension, coronary heart disease, cerebrovascular disease, and diabetes. This issue has gained increasing recognition. Excessive alcohol intake can cause emotional agitation, rapid heart rate, and increased blood pressure. It can lead to acute alcohol poisoning, acute gastric mucosal damage, and may trigger acute pancreatitis, angina, acute myocardial infarction, a surge in blood pressure, cerebral hemorrhage, acute liver failure, and sudden death.

Lack of Exercise

More than 2,400 years ago, Hippocrates, regarded as the "Father of Medicine," told people that "sunlight, air, water, and exercise are the sources of life and health." It has long been proven that individuals who lack exercise have higher incidences of hypertension, coronary heart disease, cerebrovascular disease, diabetes, and obesity. Studies have also shown that once atherosclerosis develops, current medical science cannot reverse it, but moderate exercise can cause a reversal. Additionally, I have rescued patients with pulmonary embolism on multiple occasions, most of whom had a sedentary lifestyle.

Prolonged sitting impairs venous return, creating conditions conducive to thrombus formation, leading to deep vein thrombosis in the legs. Once a clot dislodges, it can travel through the bloodstream to the pulmonary artery, resulting in pulmonary embolism and possibly sudden death. Therefore, I recommend that those who work long hours in front of a computer or have other sedentary jobs should stand up and move every 40-50 minutes, or at most every hour. Stretch your arms and legs, move your head and neck, do squats, or even simple exercises at your desk. If you are too busy, you can still move while seated, such as alternately lifting your heels and toes to activate your calf muscles and promote venous return in the legs, reducing the risk of deep vein thrombosis and pulmonary embolism. You can also stretch your upper body, rub your face and eyes to reduce fatigue.

■ Staying Up Late for Long Periods

Staying up late doesn't just cost you sleep—it can cost you your life. People should align with their body's natural biological clock. Medical research shows that chronic sleep deprivation is associated with the development of 19 diseases, including cancer, obesity, Alzheimer's, Parkinson's, neurosis, memory loss, weakened immunity, gastrointestinal disorders, diabetes, hypertension, coronary heart disease, cerebrovascular disease, and sudden death.

It has been proven that many young people, after long periods of staying up late, excessive online activity, or extreme overtime, ultimately suffer the tragedy of sudden death.

One particular situation to highlight is staying up late to watch sports. Every major sporting event, there are cases of fans suffering sudden death. Though the overall incidence is low, it's worth noting that the rate peaks during major events like the World Cup or the UEFA European Championship.

Learn New First-Aid Skills

Avoid sudden death by making small changes in your daily life.

Category	Description
Quit Smoking	The likelihood of smokers developing coronary heart disease is 2 to 10 times higher than non-smokers. Smoking is the leading risk factor for myocardial infarction and cardiovascular disease, especially for younger individuals.
Healthy Diet	Avoid the "three high" diet — high fat, high salt, high sugar. Avoid excessive alcohol consumption.
Moderate Exercise	Moderate exercise can reverse atherosclerosis and prevent cardiovascular diseases, reducing the incidence of sudden death.
Regular Routine, Less Staying Up Late	Prolonged late-night work and insufficient sleep are associated with the occurrence of 19 diseases, including sudden death. Staying up late doesn't just cost you sleep, it can cost you your life.

Emergency Scene

One night, we were dispatched to rescue a patient. We arrived at the scene in less than 10 minutes. The patient, a man in his fifties, was lying face down on the ground, unconscious, with blue lips and face, dilated pupils, and his corneas had already lost their luster. His heart had stopped beating, and he wasn't breathing. We immediately began cardiac monitoring, and the machine showed a flatline. The TV was still on, showing an intense football match.

This was a family of four. While we were performing resuscitation, we asked about the patient's medical history. The family replied, "About 20 minutes ago, he was watching the match, yelling and shouting in excitement. We told him, 'Keep your voice down, why are you yelling?' but he didn't listen. Then, all of a sudden, he shouted, 'Great goal, it's in!' Right after that, he collapsed to the ground and didn't respond no matter how we called him. His face turned purple, and he wasn't breathing. We were so scared, and it took us a while to realize what was happening. Only then did we think to call

120."

Clearly, his heart and breathing had already stopped for over 20 minutes, meaning he had already experienced brain death. We continued the resuscitation for more than 30 minutes, but the patient showed no signs of response, and unfortunately, we couldn't save him.

Of course, there are many other known risk factors. In modern society, with high levels of stress, we need to advocate for a healthy, scientific lifestyle that includes a balanced diet, moderate exercise, quitting smoking and limiting alcohol, and maintaining mental well-being to keep the hidden dangers of sudden death at bay.

What is Exercise-Induced Sudden Death?

Exercise-induced sudden death refers to unexpected death occurring during exercise or within 6-12 hours after exercise. It is similar to the general medical definition of sudden death, with the primary difference being that it happens during or shortly after physical activity. The time from the onset of symptoms to death is typically extremely short, often only seconds or minutes, which is the most critical characteristic of exercise-induced sudden death.

In recent years, sudden deaths have occurred in almost every marathon race. In 2015 alone, five cases of exercise-induced sudden death were reported in domestic marathons. Some participants, running a long-distance race for the first time, collapsed midway through the race and died suddenly. Despite being rushed to the hospital, they couldn't be saved due to delayed rescue. In some cases, although the person received defibrillation and CPR from rescue personnel, the efforts were still unsuccessful, and they died.

On October 25, 2015, during the Hefei International Marathon, a male participant in the half-marathon event suddenly collapsed near the finish line. On-site medical staff immediately performed CPR and artificial respiration, but he remained unconscious and unresponsive. He was rushed to the nearest hospital, but despite four hours of intensive resuscitation efforts, the participant sadly passed away.

This shows how urgent and dangerous exercise-induced sudden death can be.

Marathon racing is a high-load, high-intensity, long-distance, and high-risk sport, requiring athletes to be in excellent physical condition. Participants must undergo systematic training and gradually build their endurance. Before competing, they should undergo comprehensive physical examinations. If any health concerns arise, they should not participate. Individuals with heart disease, hypertension, diabetes, colds, obesity, or advanced age should also avoid marathon competitions.

The incidence of exercise-induced sudden death is 0.25 to 2.3 per 100,000 people, with the highest risk among individuals aged 30 to 50. It occurs primarily in sports like soccer, tennis, cycling, athletics, swimming, basketball, and even during physical education classes. Most people who experience exercise-induced sudden death have pre-existing organic diseases, with cardiovascular conditions (such as coronary heart disease, coronary artery anomalies, myocarditis, heart valve disease, hypertrophic cardiomyopathy, and aortic rupture) being the most common cause. Cerebrovascular accidents are another frequent culprit. Additionally, respiratory system conditions like exercise-induced asthma, pulmonary embolism, and primary pulmonary hypertension can also be triggered or worsened by exercise and lead to death if not promptly recognized and treated.

The "Extreme Point" in Long-Distance Running

Many long-distance runners experience what is known as the "extreme point," a point where the body feels extremely uncomfortable. Symptoms include a rapid heartbeat, chest tightness, difficulty breathing, feelings of suffocation, dizziness, pale complexion, cold sweats, physical exhaustion, nausea, and vomiting. At this point, many runners may consider giving up. This typically happens midway through the race or during the final sprint. Well-trained athletes can usually push through this "extreme point," but those who don't run regularly are more likely to face accidents during this stage. To avoid incidents, runners should slow down gradually when they reach the "extreme point" and only speed up once their bodies have adjusted. Otherwise, they are at high risk of experiencing events like exercise-induced sudden death.

What to Do If Someone Experiences Exercise-Induced Sudden Death?

If a participant suffers exercise-induced sudden death during a race, rescuers should immediately lay the patient flat and begin chest compressions while notifying emergency medical personnel. Using an AED (Automated External Defibrillator) to perform a cardiac shock as quickly as possible is essential.

This brings to mind the March 15, 2015, Wuxi International Marathon. This race marked the first successful use of an AED to rescue a patient during a marathon in China. It was a remarkable event that raised awareness about the importance of AEDs.

During the race, a participant suddenly collapsed. The emergency team quickly arrived and confirmed that the person had stopped breathing. One rescuer immediately began chest compressions, while others rushed to get the AED. Three minutes later, the AED was applied, and the runner's heartbeat, breathing, and consciousness were gradually restored, saving his life. Similar successful rescues occurred in the 2016 Hainan International Marathon and the Shanghai Songjiang Half Marathon in 2016, where timely CPR and AED use saved lives after participants experienced sudden death.

Life or Death: The "Golden 4 Minutes"

From a medical standpoint, the first four minutes after a sudden cardiac arrest are critical for saving a life. If someone can perform effective CPR during this period, it significantly increases the chances of survival. This time frame is known as the "golden 4 minutes."

In 2007, a survey in the Pudong district of Shanghai revealed that only 11.6% of 12,000 citizens were aware of the importance of the "golden 4 minutes."

When sudden cardiac arrest occurs, all tissues and organs in the body are damaged to varying degrees, with brain tissue being the most affected. The brain consumes the most oxygen of any organ in the body. Although it accounts for only 2% of the body's weight, it receives 15% of the body's blood flow and consumes 20-30% of its oxygen supply (and up to 50% in infants).

Therefore, the brain tissue is more vulnerable to oxygen deprivation than any other organ and is the most sensitive to a lack of oxygen. If a hand is severed, with its blood and oxygen supply completely cut off, as long as the conditions are favorable—such as a clean cut, keeping the severed limb dry, and preserving it at a low temperature—the hand can typically be reattached successfully within 3 hours. However, for brain tissue, the time it can endure a lack of blood and oxygen cannot be measured in hours but rather in minutes and seconds.

Usually, after a cardiac arrest, the patient may present with the following symptoms in chronological order:

Time Interval	Description
Immediate	Loss of heart sound, pulse, and blood pressure.
3–4 seconds	Dizziness, vision blurring, and nausea occur.
10–20 seconds	Due to severe brain hypoxia, the patient loses consciousness suddenly, possibly with whole-body convulsions and tonic-clonic seizures. The pupils are fixed and dilated, the face turns pale, and lips

Time Interval	Description
	become cyanotic.
30–40 seconds	Pupils dilate, and the light reflex disappears.
40–60 seconds	Breathing stops or presents as gasping, potentially accompanied by loss of bladder and bowel control. However, if cardiac arrest is caused by choking, drowning, or other asphyxiating causes, the patient may experience different reactions, with breathing ceasing first, followed by cardiac arrest.

If the heart and breathing stop for more than 4 to 6 minutes, irreversible damage to the brain tissue will occur! Even if the person is revived, it's hard to avoid leaving behind aftereffects. The mildest aftereffect may be sluggish responses and memory loss, while the most severe could result in a vegetative state. Of course, there are varying degrees of aftereffects between these two extremes, leading to permanent regret. If the heart and breathing stop for more than 10 minutes, brain death occurs, and the person becomes unsalvageable.

Therefore, it is crucial to begin rescue within 4 to 6 minutes. The earlier the rescue starts, the higher the success rate of resuscitation, and the fewer the aftereffects. For every minute of delay, the rescue success rate drops by 10%.

Emergency Rescue Scene

1.

Many people have heard or seen news reports about vehicles deliberately blocking ambulances. Some treat it as a joke, listening or watching without understanding the severity of such behavior. I have personally encountered several such incidents. The most dramatic one happened when we were dispatched to an alley to rescue an elderly woman who suddenly suffered from severe chest pain.

That day, when our ambulance reached Di'anmen Street, a man driving a yellow sedan, for some reason, decided to play a prank on us.

He blocked our way and intentionally drove slowly. We used the siren, but he still didn't give way. We tried changing lanes several times to bypass him, but he immediately switched lanes to block us again. Later, the driver stuck his head out of the window; he was a young man who even made faces at us. At that moment, I was so furious that I wanted to yell at him.

What should have been a 5-minute trip was extended to over 10 minutes. Finally, the yellow sedan stopped at the entrance to the alley we were heading to. Since we were in a rush to save the patient, we didn't have time to argue with him. We quickly got out of the vehicle and ran toward the scene. To our surprise, the young man was headed the same way. As we entered the courtyard, we heard crying from a room. The young man's face suddenly changed, and he ran into the house ahead of us. We followed him in. An elderly woman was lying on the ground, surrounded by people crying and questioning us: "Why are you so late?" I pointed to the young man who had just entered and said, "Ask him." He didn't say a word.

We examined the patient and found that the elderly woman had already stopped breathing and had no heartbeat. At that moment, the young man began wailing, "Mom, it's all my fault…" Seeing him in such agony, we were both angry and sympathetic. Despite our best efforts to revive her, it was too late. If the elderly woman's own son hadn't blocked the ambulance, we could have arrived a few minutes earlier, and his mother might not have died. I don't believe in karma, but this coincidence was too much.

Of course, the final outcome of the rescue depends on many factors, with the two most important being the severity of the condition and whether the rescue is timely and correct.

I have shared these heartbreaking examples to emphasize that the next person who experiences sudden death might be you, me, or our family or friends. Everyone should learn some basic first aid knowledge to save themselves or others in critical moments.

2.
Now, let me tell you two more stories, both

coincidentally involving foreigners.

The first story happened over 10 years ago.

One day, Sony Ericsson in Shunyi District, Beijing, invited me through the Red Cross Society of Chongwen District (now part of Dongcheng District) to conduct first aid training. Before the training began, an employee of the company shared a true story with me: On the evening of April 8, 2004, at 6:30 p.m., the 54-year-old president of Ericsson (China), Mr. Jan Maij, a former reserve officer of the Swedish Royal Air Force, suddenly died of a heart attack at the company's reception desk (contrary to online reports claiming he died on a treadmill). It was after work hours, and although many people were around, no one helped him. By the time doctors arrived, he was already dead. Why didn't anyone help? Because everyone present was Chinese, and none of them knew how to perform CPR!

This is a deeply frustrating story. Every time I give lectures, I reflect on it: Firstly, if this Swedish man had suffered a sudden death in

Sweden, he likely would have been saved, as Sweden had one of the highest CPR awareness rates in the world at the time. Secondly, I lament the fact that too few people in China knew CPR back then. Later, after Ericsson and Sony merged to form Sony Ericsson, their company bus was involved in an accident, resulting in over 20 casualties. Mr. Maij's sudden death, coupled with the bus accident, prompted the company leadership to decide on first aid training for all employees. I went there for several years, at least twice a year, and the company became one of the most committed to learning first aid in the Beijing area.

Why wait until someone dies to learn first aid? You should learn it during normal times to be prepared for emergencies.

3.

The second story is a heartwarming one that took place at the Shangri-La Hotel near Zizhuyuan Bridge.

Because I often conducted first aid training at major hotels in Beijing, I became good friends with Manager Xiao from the Health Department and Dr. Qu from the hotel's medical office. The staff at the hotel also became familiar with me.

That day, as soon as I entered the hotel, two female staff members greeted me excitedly: "Teacher Jia, a few days ago, we saved a foreign guest who had a sudden cardiac arrest." I said, "Really? You're not exaggerating, are you?" Other staff members chimed in, "It's true! If you don't believe us, ask Dr. Zhang from your 120 emergency team; he was the one who came to rescue that day."

Later, when I returned to the emergency center, I checked the records and found that Dr. Zhang Shuangsen had indeed gone to Shangri-La that day. I asked him, "A few days ago, you went to Shangri-La and successfully resuscitated a foreigner?" Dr. Zhang replied, "Yes, but it was thanks to the hotel staff's timely efforts. Our vehicle wasn't far away, but we got stuck in traffic. We rushed there as quickly as we could, but it still took over 10 minutes. When we arrived, the patient had no heartbeat or breathing, and the staff was kneeling beside him, performing

CPR. I said, 'They're doing a pretty good job.' They told me, 'It was your Teacher Jia who taught us.' I was just about to administer medication and hook up the heart monitor, but before I could start the rescue, the patient's heartbeat and breathing had already returned! If they hadn't acted first, by the time we arrived, it would have been too late." After further professional care from Dr. Zhang, the patient quickly regained consciousness, making it a successful resuscitation case.

The reason this foreign guest was able to come back to life was primarily due to the hotel staff's timely and correct first aid, and, of course, Dr. Zhang Shuangsen's rich experience in resuscitation.

———

From these two contrasting stories, it's clear that two factors are crucial to a patient's survival: the importance of the 4 to 6-minute window, also known as the "golden 4 minutes" for sudden cardiac arrest, and whether the patient receives timely and correct first aid during that critical period.

However, no matter how fast an ambulance is, it's often impossible to reach the patient within minutes. No matter how advanced the hospital equipment is, or how skilled the doctors are, most patients cannot be transported to the hospital within minutes. So, are we just waiting for death? Is there a solution? Yes! The patient and those around them must provide immediate assistance, buying time and creating conditions for the arrival of the ambulance. You must seize the "golden 4 minutes" of rescue.

Therefore, in addition to promoting a healthy lifestyle to prevent and reduce the occurrence of diseases and sudden death, learning CPR is the best way to respond to sudden death! If at least one or two people in every family learn CPR, the tragedies of sudden death would greatly decrease. After calling 120, you wouldn't be left helpless.

Everyone Should Learn CPR: Equip Yourself with Life-Saving Skills

After discussing sudden death and emergency rescue at length, the most important thing for each of us to learn is cardiopulmonary resuscitation (CPR). This is a life-saving technique that can revive a sudden cardiac arrest victim in a critical situation, and it requires no medical equipment or specialized knowledge. As long as you have hands and follow the correct procedure, you can perform CPR. In many of the cases mentioned earlier, if even one person around the patient knew CPR and provided timely aid before the ambulance arrived, the patient might have survived.

In developed countries like those in Europe and the U.S., CPR is one of the basic skills nearly everyone is expected to learn. In the 1990s, the United States passed legislation to implement the "Public Access Defibrillation" program, which installed Automated External Defibrillators (AEDs) in public places. The goal was to ensure AEDs could be accessed within 10 minutes, and regular people were trained in how to use them.

What is CPR?

CPR (Cardiopulmonary Resuscitation) refers to a series of emergency measures taken to restore the heart, breathing, and brain function of a patient experiencing sudden cardiac arrest. These measures include manual chest compressions, rescue breathing, and the use of related equipment like AEDs.

Let's Learn a New Life-Saving Skill: CPR in 7 Steps for Adults

1. Assess the Safety of the Scene
2. Check if the Patient is Conscious and Breathing
3. Call Emergency Services Immediately
4. Place the Patient in the Recovery Position
5. Chest Compressions (Circulation)
6. Open the Airway (Airway)
7. Perform Rescue Breathing (Breathing)

CPR for Newborns

1. Open the Airway (A)
2. Rescue Breathing (Mouth-to-Mouth and Nose)
(B)
3. Chest Compressions (C)

For adults, the CPR sequence is generally CAB (Circulation, Airway, Breathing), while for newborns, it follows ABC (Airway, Breathing, Circulation).

Step 1: Assess the Safety of the Scene

Before entering the scene, the rescuer must first observe and understand the overall environment. The scene can often provide clues about the nature of the incident, the injuries that have occurred, and the potential dangers that could continue to cause harm. Take necessary protective measures and eliminate any threats before entering. Only when the rescuer's own safety is ensured can they begin rescuing the patient. Otherwise, the situation could worsen, potentially causing even greater harm. In addition to calling 120, emergency services, it may also be necessary to request help from specialized personnel, such as firefighters or rescue engineers.

Step 2: Check if the Patient is Conscious and Breathing

The rescuer should gently tap the patient's shoulders and call out loudly. If there is no response, observe the chest for 5 to 10 seconds to determine whether the patient is breathing by checking for chest movement.

Step 3: Call Emergency Services Immediately

If the patient is unconscious and not breathing, call 120 to contact emergency medical services and get professional help as soon as possible. If others are present at the scene, ask them to make the call quickly. In cases of drowning, trauma, poisoning, or for children under 8 years old, perform CPR for 5 cycles (about 2 minutes) before calling for help (you can use the speakerphone function on your phone to call while continuing CPR).

If there are two people present at the rescue scene, one should immediately call 120 while the other starts performing CPR and tries to obtain an AED.

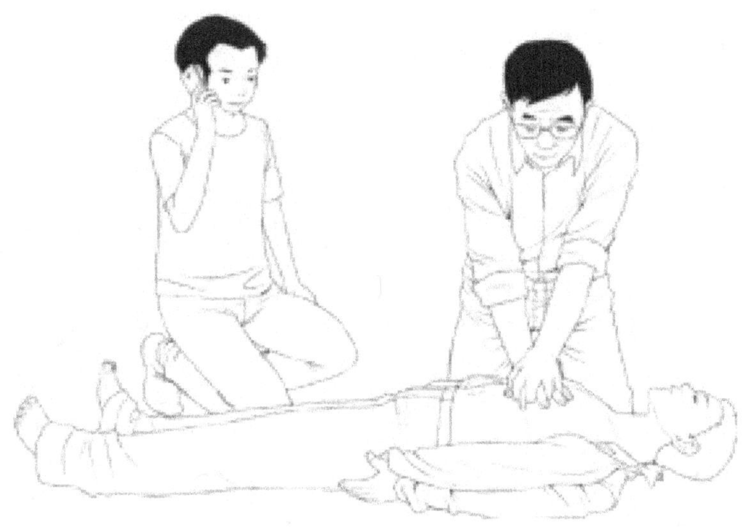

Step 4: Place the Patient in the Supine Position for Resuscitation

The "recovery position" here refers to the supine position (lying on the back). If the patient is not already in this position, the rescuer should place them on their back. However, this must be done carefully and following a specific procedure to avoid causing further injury.

1. Kneel beside the patient's body and extend both of their arms straight up above their head. Position the far leg over the near leg, crossing them at the knees.

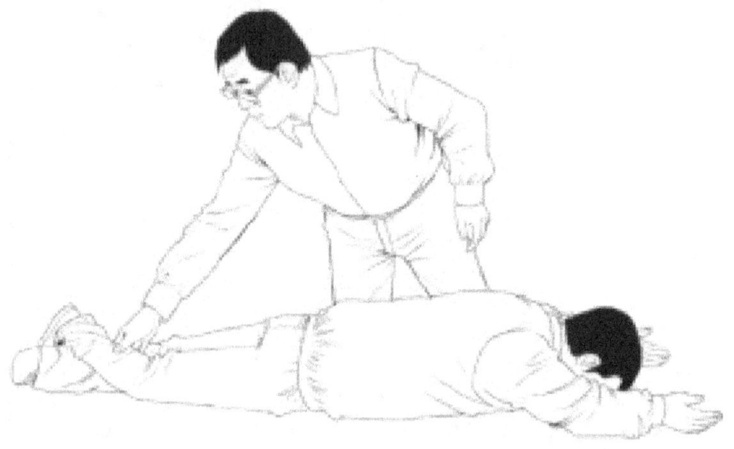

2. The patient's head, neck, waist, and hips must be aligned along the same axis, avoiding any twisting or bending of the body. This ensures that the body remains in a straight line to prevent further injury.

3.

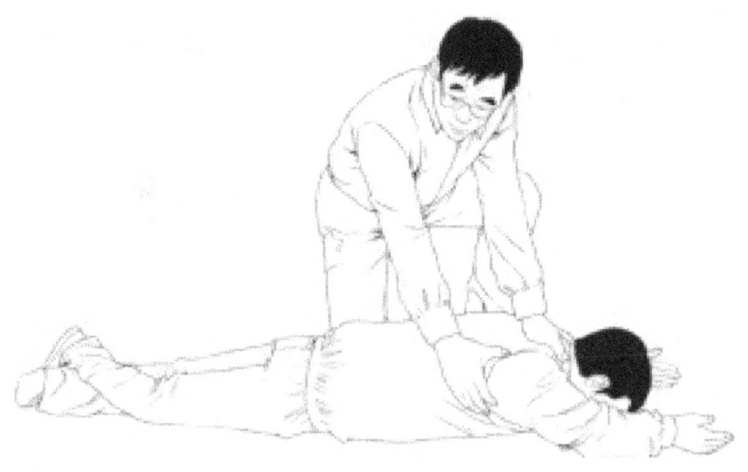

4. Place one hand on the back of the patient's neck to stabilize it, and the other hand under the far-side armpit. Then, using firm pressure, carefully roll the patient as a whole into the supine position.

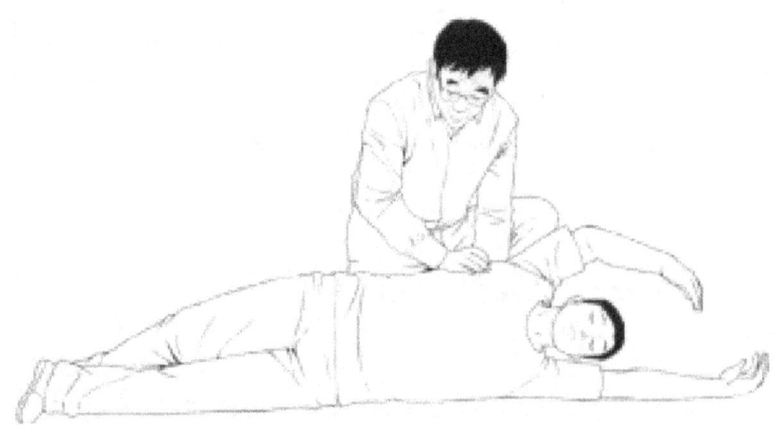

5. The patient's head should not be elevated

above the chest, and nothing should be placed under the head.

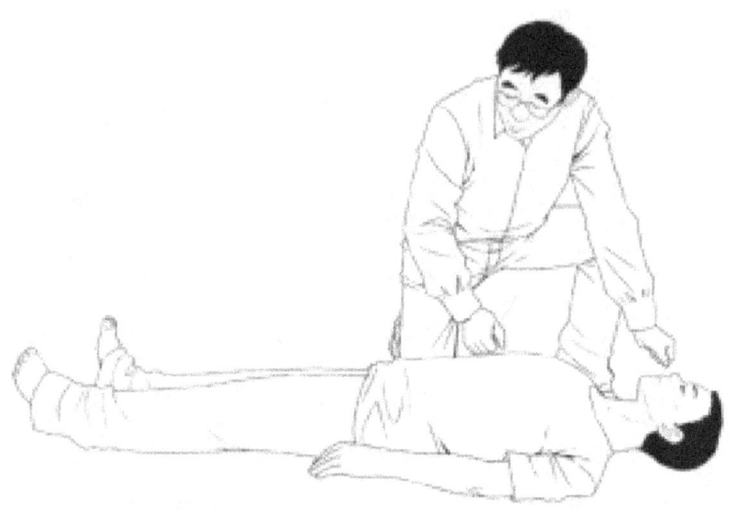

The surface where the patient is lying should be firm, not on a soft bed or couch. If the surface is too soft, chest compressions may not be deep enough, reducing the effectiveness of the compressions and the heart's ability to pump blood.

Step 5: Chest Compressions

Chest compressions are the most crucial step in CPR, as they help restore circulation in the body. When done correctly, they can achieve 25-30% of the heart's normal blood output, and the brain's blood flow can reach about 30% of its normal level.

First, the rescuer should kneel beside the patient, with knees apart and shoulder-width. Position your body directly over the patient's nipple line. Using your hips as the pivot point, press straight down on the patient's sternum, utilizing the weight of your upper body and the strength of your shoulders and arms.

Important! Keep both arms straight at all times, with your hands perpendicular to the ground during compressions. Avoid leaning, tilting, or bending your arms, and ensure your body does not sway. Maintaining this form is essential to ensure the effectiveness of the compressions.

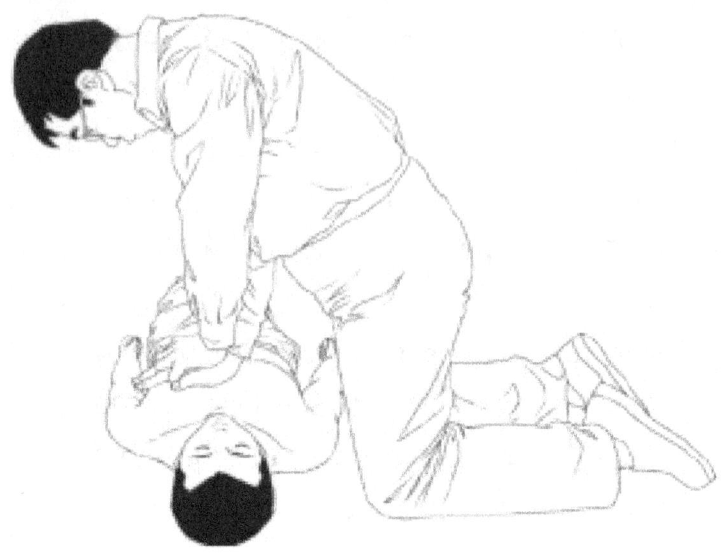

Secondly, the selection of the compression site is crucial. In principle, you should aim for the lower half of the patient's sternum. Place the heel of one hand on the midpoint of the line connecting the two nipples, ensuring it is centered and not off to the side. Your middle finger should be aligned with the far nipple. Then, place your other hand on top, overlapping with the first hand, with both heels of your palms aligned. Interlock your fingers to ensure the heels of your palms remain in the center of the sternum.

During compressions, the heel of your hand must stay in constant contact with the chest wall to prevent the compression site from shifting.

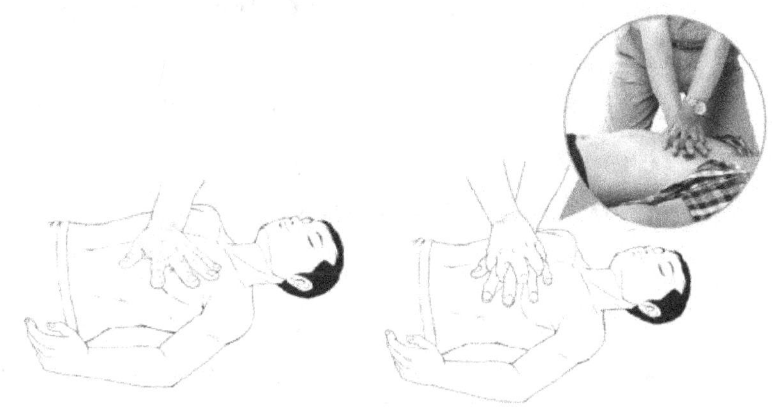

How deep should the compressions be for them to be effective?

The compression depth should be 5 to 6 centimeters or depress the chest wall by about one-third of its thickness. Ideally, you should be able to feel the carotid pulse during compressions.

The compression rate should be between 100 and 120 times per minute.

During compressions, when you allow your hands to relax, ensure that the heel of your hand remains in contact with the patient's chest wall to allow for complete recoil of the chest. This is crucial; if the chest wall does not fully rebound, it can reduce venous return and negatively impact the effectiveness of the resuscitation.

Step 6: Open the Airway

Why is this step necessary? When a person loses consciousness, especially after cardiac arrest, their overall muscle tone decreases, including the muscles in the throat and tongue. This loss of muscle tone can cause the tongue to fall back, potentially leading to airway obstruction and hindering breathing.

To prevent this, it's essential to ensure that the airway is open, allowing for adequate airflow during resuscitation efforts.

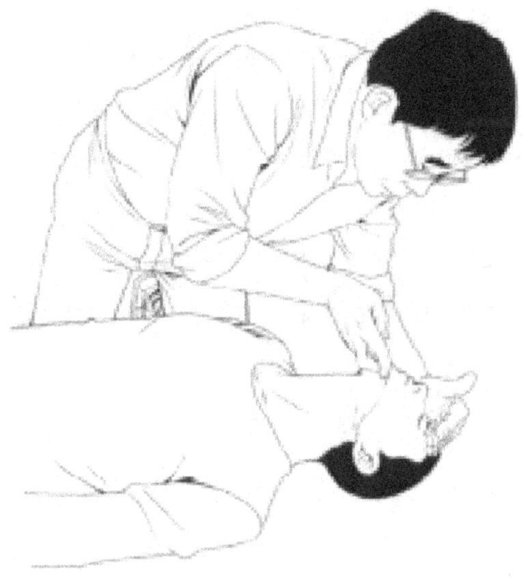

How to Open the Airway?

Use the "Head-Tilt, Chin-Lift" maneuver: Place the heel of one hand on the patient's forehead and apply gentle pressure downward. With the fingers of your other hand (index and middle fingers) together, place them under the bony part of the patient's chin and lift it upward. This will elevate the chin and lower jaw while tilting the head back. The line between the earlobe and the angle of the jaw should be perpendicular to the surface on which the patient is lying (i.e., the nostrils should be facing directly upward). This position opens the airway.

Step 7: Rescue Breathing (Mouth-to-Mouth)

After opening the airway, use your index and middle fingers to pinch the patient's nostrils shut. Then, seal your mouth tightly around the patient's mouth and provide two breaths into their lungs. Make sure to deliver each breath steadily and fully.

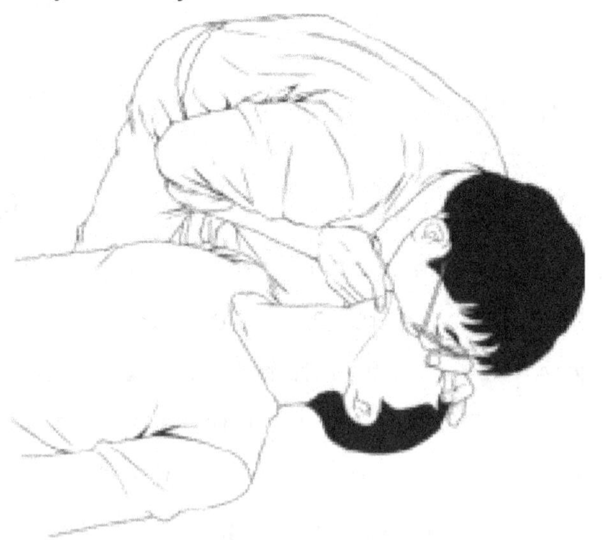

After each breath, turn your head to the side to breathe in, and then release your fingers from pinching the patient's nostrils before delivering the second breath. Each breath should last about 1 second; it should not be too long or too forceful. You should see the patient's chest rise visibly.

If the breaths are too forceful or prolonged, it can lead to gastric inflation and increased pressure in the abdomen, which compresses the lungs and reduces ventilation. Additionally, it may cause the stomach contents to regurgitate into the mouth, potentially leading to airway obstruction.

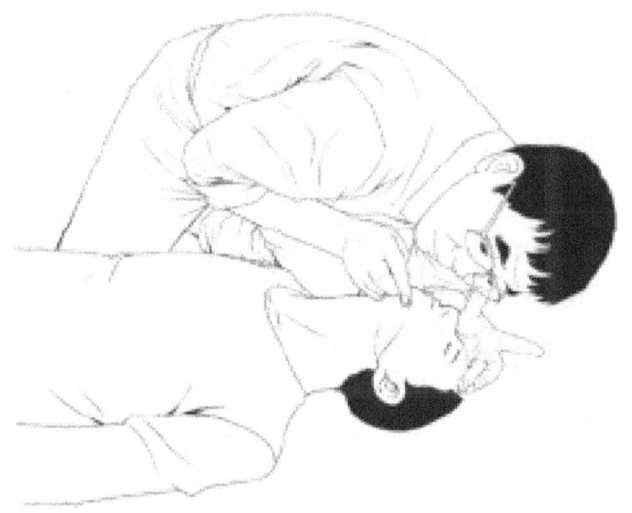

Typically, the ratio of chest compressions to rescue breaths is 30:2. This means that for every 30 compressions, you should provide 2 rescue breaths. This sequence continues until an AED (Automated External Defibrillator) is available for use or emergency personnel arrive to take over.

After 5 cycles (approximately 2 minutes), check the patient's pulse. To check the carotid pulse, rotate the patient's neck to identify the prominent muscle that runs from the ear to the sternum, known as the sternocleidomastoid muscle. You can feel the carotid pulse by placing your index and middle fingers horizontally on the thyroid cartilage and then sliding them to the edge of the sternocleidomastoid muscle.

If a pulse is detected, it indicates that the heart has restarted, and you should stop compressions. If no pulse is felt, continue with the compressions and check the pulse every 5 minutes thereafter.

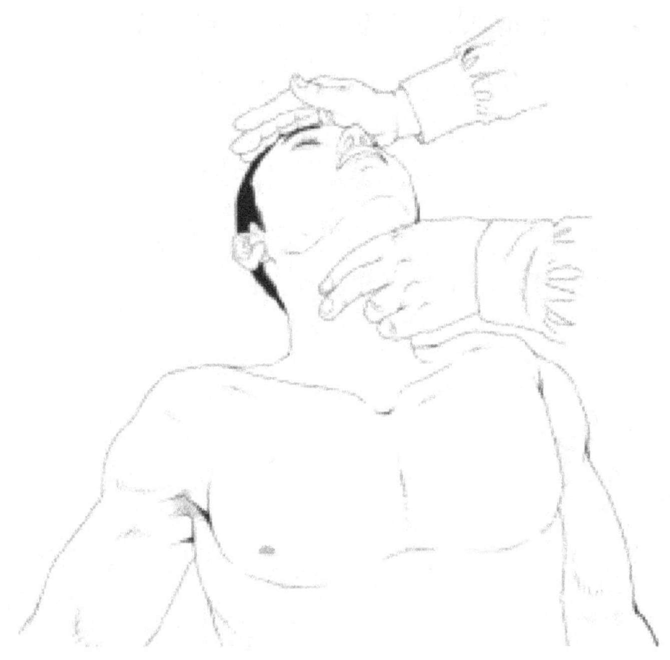

I would like to point out that many medical rescue practices depicted in domestic films and TV dramas are incorrect. For example, in some dramas, when a rescuer sees a victim lying on the ground, they often check for a pulse by feeling the radial artery at the wrist. This practice is misguided because the absence of a radial pulse does not necessarily indicate that the heart has stopped beating. The most reliable method to determine if the heart has stopped is by checking for a pulse in the carotid artery.

It is also important to note that infants have underdeveloped systems, and their CPR procedures differ significantly from those for adults. When assessing an infant's level of consciousness, one effective method is to stimulate the soles of their feet.

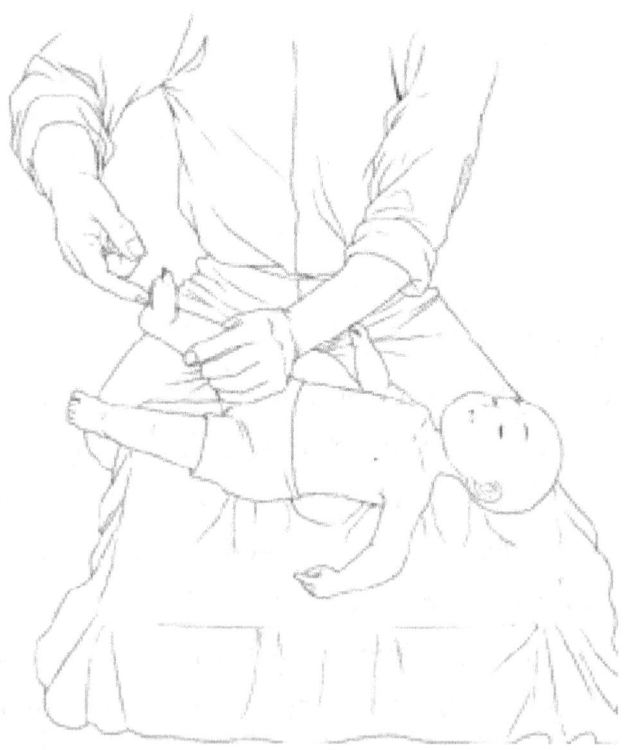

To determine whether an infant has a heartbeat, you can check the brachial artery.

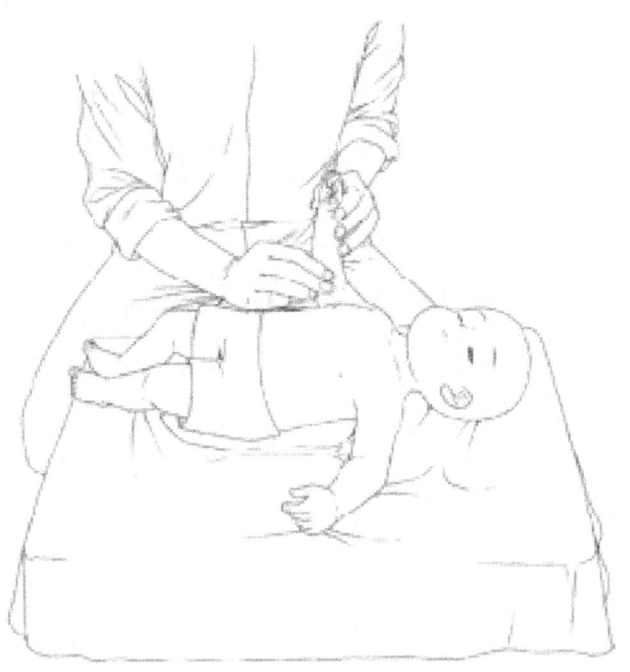

You can also assess an infant's heartbeat by checking the femoral artery.

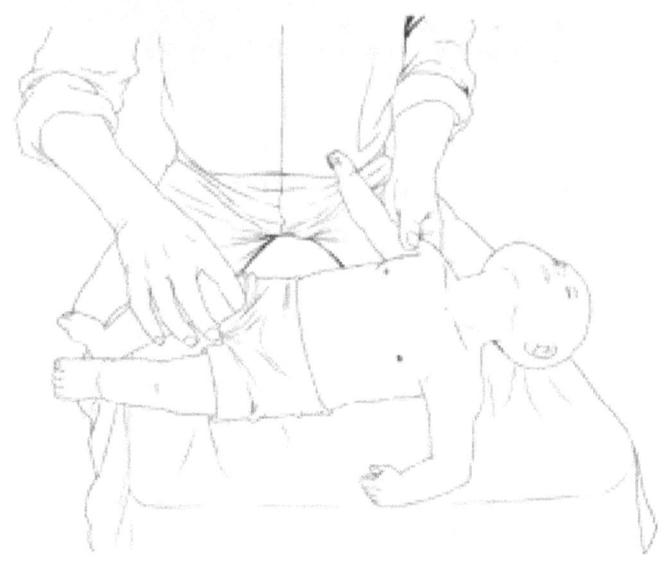

The compression site for infants is located directly below the midpoint of the line connecting the two nipples. Typically, use the two-finger technique for compressions. Place the index and middle fingers of one hand together, with the fingertips pressing down vertically. The compression depth should be about one-third of the infant's chest wall thickness, and the rate should be between 100 and 120 compressions per minute.

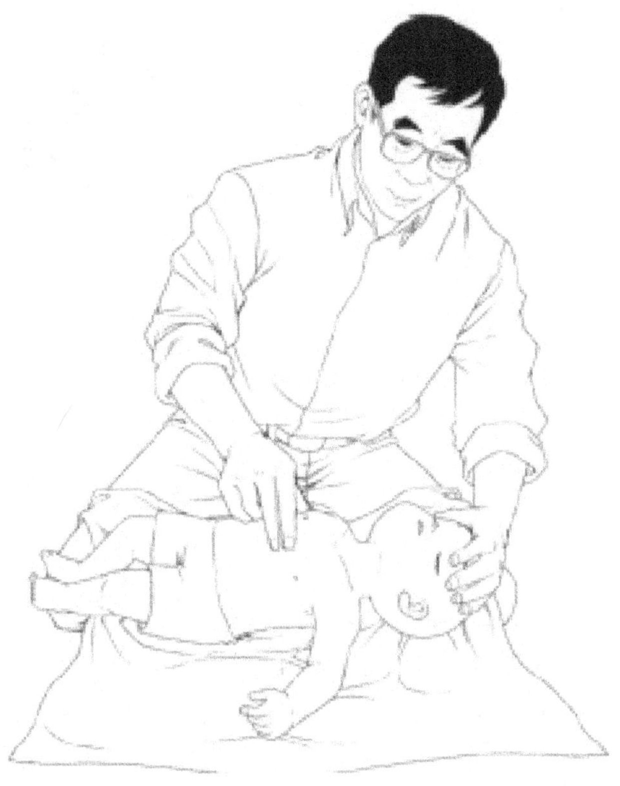

Additionally, when opening the airway for an infant, the line connecting the angle of the jaw to the earlobe should be at a 30° angle to the surface on which the infant is lying. During rescue breathing, it is sufficient to observe visible rise and fall of the chest wall to confirm that air is entering the lungs.

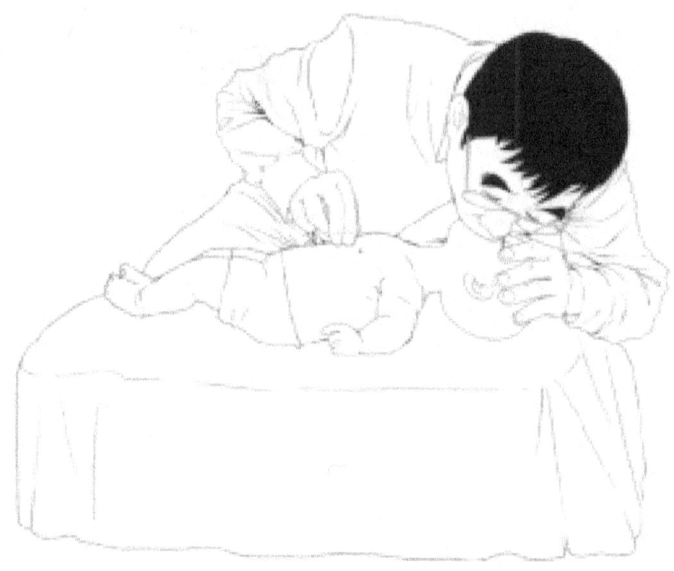

In the case of newborns experiencing cardiac arrest, the order of resuscitation follows the ABC sequence: Airway, Breathing, and Chest Compressions. While the content of CPR can be extensive, we can summarize the key points of CPR into the "Four Steps of CPR": Assess—Call 120—Compress—Defibrillate.

Currently, for the vast majority of people in China, the lack of AED devices means they can only perform the first three steps, and most people may only manage to do two. The next person who may suffer from sudden cardiac arrest could be you, me, or our loved ones. It is my hope that these two steps can be expanded to three, or even four.

Time is life; life is in your hands. Learning CPR can save precious lives.

Comparison of the key points of cardiopulmonary resuscitation in adults, children and infants:

	Adult	Child	Infant
Chest Compression Position	Center of the line between the nipples	Center of the line between the nipples	Just below the center of the line between the nipples
Compression Method	Both hands (heel of the palm)	One hand (heel of the palm)	Two fingers (index and middle fingers)
Compression Rate	100–120 times/min	At least 100–120 times/min but not more than	Same as child

	Adult	Child	Infant
Compression Depth	5–6 cm	140 times/min 1/3 to 1/2 of chest depth	1/3 to 1/2 of chest depth
Artificial Respiration Method	Mouth-to-mouth	Mouth-to-mouth	Mouth-to-nose or mouth-to-mouth
Compression-to-Breath Ratio	30:2	30:2 (single rescuer), 15:2 (two rescuers)	15:2

Life-Saving Device: AED

Emergency Scene

On March 21, 2015, my friend, Professor Tang Ziren, Deputy Director of the Emergency Department at Beijing Chaoyang Hospital, was visiting SeaWorld in San Diego when an

American tourist suddenly collapsed about 10 meters away from him due to cardiac arrest. Professor Tang performed chest compressions alone for over 10 minutes until an AED arrived, after which the tourist was successfully resuscitated! The park management was extremely grateful and offered him a complimentary meal where he could watch a private whale show to make up for missing the performance.

Afterward, Professor Tang admitted, "If there had been no AED at the time, I might not have been able to save her." This wasn't modesty or politeness—it was the truth.

At 7:30 PM on June 29, 2016, Mr. Jin Bo, Deputy Editor-in-Chief of Tianya Community, suddenly collapsed at the Hujialou Station on Beijing's Subway Line 6 while on his way home from work. Several bystanders voluntarily performed CPR on him, and subway staff called for an ambulance. Sadly, despite their efforts, the 34-year-old Jin Bo did not survive.

Mr. Jin Bo's sudden death sparked

unprecedented public attention and widespread discussions about AEDs. In China, AEDs are not available in most crowded public places such as subway stations, train stations, airports, airplanes, trains, stadiums, hotels, large shopping malls, or emergency vehicles like police cars and fire trucks. This has become a major public health concern.

To understand AEDs, we must first explain what ventricular fibrillation is.

Ventricular Fibrillation (VF) is short for ventricular fibrillation, a condition in which the heart's ventricular muscles contract rapidly and weakly or in a disorganized manner. This results in the heart losing its ability to pump blood, causing the pulse, heart sounds, and blood pressure to disappear. Blood flow to the heart, brain, and other organs is completely interrupted. VF is a fatal heart rhythm disorder that leads to sudden death.

After cardiac arrest, more than 80% of cases show VF on an electrocardiogram within the first 3–5 minutes. The only effective way to treat VF is through defibrillation.

The sooner defibrillation is performed, the higher the success rate. If defibrillation is completed within 1 minute, the success rate can be as high as 90%. For every minute of delay, the success rate decreases by 10%. Timely defibrillation is key to saving lives.

So, what exactly is an AED, and how does it relate to defibrillation?
AED stands for Automated External Defibrillator. It is an emergency device specifically designed for non-medical personnel. Small, lightweight, and easy to operate, AEDs are safe to use.

In simple terms, using an AED can eliminate ventricular fibrillation, allowing the heart's sinoatrial node to resume function, thus restoring the heartbeat. AEDs are easy to master with basic training and are actually simpler to learn than manual CPR.

Rescuers only need to operate steps 1, 2, 3, and 6. Some AEDs only require steps 1, 2, and 6. If using a fully automated AED, only two steps are required: press the power button and follow the voice prompts to apply the electrode pads. The

AED will automatically analyze, charge, and deliver the shock, potentially bringing the patient back to life. It's truly remarkable!

When used, the AED will automatically analyze the heart rhythm. If the patient has a normal rhythm or the electrocardiogram shows a flatline (indicating the absence of VF), the AED will not charge, making it safe for both the patient and the rescuer.

According to recent data, the number of AEDs installed per 100,000 people in various countries is as follows:
Japan: 393.7 units
United States: 198.9 units
Australia: 44.5 units
United Kingdom: 25.6 units
Germany: 17.6 units

Learn a New Emergency Skill: How to Use an AED

AEDs come with batteries. First, press the power button, and follow the voice prompts for simple operation.

1. Press the power button to turn on the device, then follow the voice prompts.
2. "Please place the electrode pads on the patient as shown in the diagram."
3. "Please insert the plug into the socket."
4. "Do not touch the patient; the AED is analyzing the heart rhythm."
5. "Do not approach the patient; the AED is charging."
6. "Now, defibrillate. Please press the orange shock button."

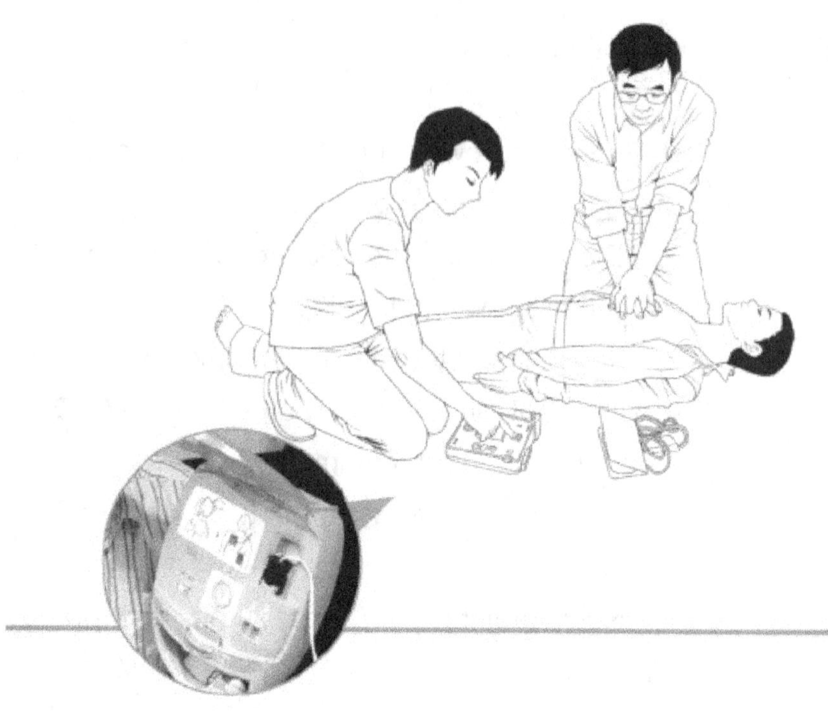

Emergency Scene

In my memory, one of the first organizations in Beijing to have an AED was the Sino-American joint venture Procter & Gamble (Beijing). I can't quite recall the exact year, but it was around 2000. A young female doctor in their medical office had asked me several times to train their employees on how to use the AED. I asked, "Who suggested equipping an AED?" She replied, "The company's boss." I asked again,

"Where is the boss from?" She answered, "The United States."

There was also an incident at the Forbidden City where a French tourist suddenly died of cardiac arrest. At that time, none of the staff knew how to perform emergency rescue, which was extremely awkward. Later, at the invitation of the Dongcheng District Red Cross, I conducted first aid training at the Forbidden City and recommended that they equip AEDs.

I have also provided emergency training for an airline multiple times. They were planning to equip all their planes and airports with AEDs. They even asked me, "How many AEDs should we place at an airport?" I answered, "It's best if an AED can reach a patient within 3 minutes. If money is not a concern, it's even better if it can be accessed within 1 minute." After that, I heard nothing more from them, so I'm not sure if they followed through with installing the AEDs. In any case, at least they became aware of the need, which is progress in itself.

For the general public in China, AEDs are not

just emergency devices, but represent a new concept of emergency rescue. Only by promoting the installation and use of AEDs, alongside widespread training in CPR techniques, can we significantly improve the success rate of CPR in the country.

In light of this, Mr. Deng Fei, Editorial Board Member and Director of the Journalism Department at Phoenix Weekly, in collaboration with institutions such as Tianya Community, Sina Weibo's Micro Charity, and Tencent Volunteers Association, has launched the "Heart Awakening" fund with the China Social Welfare Foundation. This fund, named in honor of Jin Bo, will place emergency rescue equipment, including AEDs, in public places like subways, stations, airports, and malls across major cities in China. The goal is to establish a rapid response system specifically for cardiac arrest patients. At the same time, they advocate for and promote regular professional training for staff in these locations, with the ultimate goal of making AEDs and emergency rescue systems mandatory in public places.

Since the mid-1980s, I have worked tirelessly to raise public awareness of emergency response and promote first aid knowledge and skills across society. In the late 1990s, I also began to heavily promote the installation and use of AEDs, though with limited success.

Now, I am honored to be one of the co-founders of Mr. Deng Fei's "Heart Awakening" fund. He has accomplished something that I have long dreamed of achieving but was unable to realize. I hope that through the "Heart Awakening" fund, more people will learn how to perform first aid and self-rescue. In critical moments, they will be able to help themselves or others, benefiting many lives.

Six 80% Facts about Sudden Cardiac Arrest

1. More than 80% of sudden cardiac arrests are caused by coronary heart disease.
2. More than 80% of sudden cardiac arrests occur outside of hospitals in various settings.
3. In more than 80% of sudden cardiac arrests,

the heart stops before breathing stops.

4. In more than 80% of sudden cardiac arrests, the initial heart rhythm is ventricular fibrillation.

5. More than 80% of sudden cardiac arrests are successfully resuscitated using an AED.

6. We hope that more than 80% of Chinese citizens will learn how to perform CPR and use an AED, staying safe from the threat of sudden cardiac arrest.

Chapter 2: Acute Myocardial Infarction - A Race Against Time

What Exactly is a Heart Attack?

Many people fear cancer, turning pale just at the mention of it. However, acute myocardial infarction (commonly referred to as a heart attack) is far more terrifying than cancer. Although cancer is still considered a terminal illness, even patients diagnosed with late-stage cancer usually live for a period of time. On the other hand, when someone experiences a heart attack, if they do not receive timely treatment, their life is immediately at risk. In critical cases, death can be instantaneous. Many people don't even have time to leave last words, and some may not even realize what has happened before passing away, leaving lifelong regrets for themselves and their loved ones.

In emergency medicine, some conditions are classified as emergencies, while others are considered severe illnesses. Acute myocardial infarction falls under the category of "both urgent and severe"—an extremely dangerous condition. Having worked at the Beijing Emergency Medical Center for nearly 30 years and participated in countless rescues, the most common and deadliest condition I've encountered is acute myocardial infarction. It's a race against time, where even a one-minute delay can mean the difference between life and death.

Statistics show that out of every 100 sudden deaths, 80–90 of them are caused by acute myocardial infarction. Moreover, 90% of these deaths occur outside hospitals, and most patients die within 15 minutes of the onset of the condition, with some even passing away instantly.

Emergency Scene

Once, late at night, a girl called our emergency hotline for help, saying that her father had collapsed and was unresponsive. We rushed to her home, but sadly, by the time we arrived, her father's body was already cold. We had to inform her that her father had passed away. From the time she discovered her father's condition to our arrival, less than half an hour had passed. Unfortunately, she didn't know how to perform

CPR or administer any form of first aid, and her father did not survive. Based on her description of her father's symptoms, we determined that acute myocardial infarction was likely the cause of death.

On August 8, 2014, the National Center for Cardiovascular Diseases officially released the *2013 China Cardiovascular Disease Report*, which showed that cardiovascular disease was the leading cause of death among both urban and rural residents in China, accounting for 38.7% of deaths in rural areas and 41.1% in urban areas. One in five adults suffers from cardiovascular disease, with the prevalence continuing to rise. Approximately 3.5 million people die from cardiovascular disease each year in China—that's 9,590 people per day, 400 people per hour, and one person every 10 seconds. By May 11, 2016, the National Center for Cardiovascular Diseases had released the *2015 China Cardiovascular Disease Report*, showing that in 2014, cardiovascular disease remained the leading cause of death, surpassing cancer and other diseases. Since 2009, the cardiovascular disease mortality rate in rural areas has exceeded that in urban areas. Cardiovascular disease accounts for 44.6% of all deaths in rural areas and 42.51% in cities. Nationwide, two out of every five deaths are due to cardiovascular and cerebrovascular diseases, with cerebrovascular disease being the leading cause of death for both men and women in China.

Among cardiovascular diseases, special attention must be given to coronary heart disease.

Coronary Artery Disease, also known as ischemic heart disease, occurs when atherosclerosis causes the coronary arteries to thicken and harden, narrowing or blocking the blood vessels. This leads to ischemia (reduced blood supply) or necrosis (tissue death) of the heart muscle, posing an unprecedented threat to human life and health.

Acute myocardial infarction is the most severe type of coronary heart disease. It occurs when blood flow in a coronary artery is suddenly blocked (most often due to a blood clot), causing prolonged and severe ischemia to the heart muscle, leading to its death. This condition is common among middle-aged and elderly people and is a leading cause of sudden death. Statistics show that, on average, one person dies of a heart attack every second worldwide.

Therefore, patients with coronary heart disease must be particularly vigilant and take steps to reduce the risk of acute myocardial infarction and sudden death.

You may wonder: what exactly is a "heart attack," and how does it happen?

The heart functions like a "pump" that maintains blood circulation. This pump sends blood from the heart to all organs, supplying them with oxygen and nutrients. In return, the heart itself also needs oxygen and nutrients, which are delivered through the coronary arteries.

A healthy young person has soft, elastic blood vessels with thin walls, wide lumens, and smooth inner surfaces, allowing blood to flow freely and supply oxygen to all organs. However, when cholesterol gradually deposits on the artery walls, they thicken, harden, and narrow. When these "pipes" develop problems, we call this "arteriosclerosis." Blood flow is reduced, and organs become deprived of oxygen, leading to illness.

Arteriosclerosis can occur in any artery in the body: in the brain, it's called cerebral arteriosclerosis; in the kidneys, renal arteriosclerosis. When it occurs in the coronary arteries, it's known as coronary atherosclerosis, or coronary heart disease.

Coronary heart disease's full name is coronary atherosclerotic heart disease. What does "atherosclerotic" mean? The term comes from pathology. If you were to see a cross-section of a hardened coronary artery, you would notice grayish-white, rice-porridge-like deposits on the artery walls. Pressing them, you'd find them hard. These porridge-like deposits block blood flow to the heart, and when a blood clot forms on top of them, the artery becomes completely blocked, leading to severe, prolonged ischemia and necrosis of the heart muscle, known as myocardial infarction. Once the heart muscle dies, the heart's function becomes severely impaired, putting the person's life in grave danger.

Where does this "porridge" in the arteries come from? Before the reform and opening-up period, coronary heart disease was rare in China. At that time, food was rationed, and coronary heart disease was nicknamed a "rich man's disease"—only those who could afford it suffered from it. Now, with improved living conditions and an abundance of rich, fatty foods, coupled with unhealthy lifestyles, people's arteries are increasingly filling with these "porridge-like" deposits, leading to diseases like coronary heart disease. Consequently, the incidence of acute myocardial infarction has risen.

Emergency Scene

During my nearly 30 years at the Beijing Emergency Medical Center, I encountered heart attack patients weekly. On the busiest day, I rescued four such patients. Among the countless patients I've treated, the youngest was a 23-year-old man.

This happened in the mid-1980s. The young man suddenly experienced chest pain, and his electrocardiogram showed a typical pattern of acute myocardial infarction. At first, I found it hard to believe—how could someone so young have a heart attack? After stabilizing him at the scene, I took him to Beijing Tongren Hospital. The doctors there were also unsure if it was a heart attack. Later, after checking on his condition, I confirmed that he had indeed suffered a heart attack. Fortunately, thanks to timely medical intervention, he recovered and was discharged safely.

Some might think that because heart attacks are so dangerous, it's best to stay in the hospital before any symptoms appear so you can receive immediate treatment if something goes wrong. While that would be ideal, the real danger of heart attacks lies in their unpredictability. They can strike anywhere, anytime, affecting men and women, young and old. Heart attacks often occur at night, precisely when people are least prepared and least alert.

Chest Pain: The Most Typical Warning Signal of Acute Myocardial Infarction

Since a heart attack is so dangerous, is there any way to recognize the symptoms? In fact, many patients never experience warning signs before an attack, and they often appear to be perfectly healthy. This makes such cases more dangerous because they come with no preparation—just like the father of the girl I mentioned earlier. He had never been sick before, and the family didn't even keep heart medication on hand. Statistics show that 1 in 4 coronary heart disease patients experiences sudden death during their first episode, which is a deadly threat to everyone and presents a huge challenge to medical care.

At this point, many people may be wondering: "Do I have heart disease? Could I suddenly have a heart attack one day?"

Let me explain what signals the heart might be sending out, especially the warning signs of a heart attack. Pay attention to these signs, and if you notice any of them, seek medical help immediately.

Patients may suddenly experience pain in the precordial area or behind the sternum, with the pain radiating to the shoulders, arms, or back. It may be accompanied by chest tightness and shortness of breath. The pain often feels constricting, oppressive, suffocating, or burning and may be accompanied by feelings of fear or impending doom.

The pain lasts longer than angina, often exceeding 30 minutes and can persist for several hours or even days.

Rest or sublingual nitroglycerin provides no significant relief.

Patients often experience additional symptoms such as restlessness, cyanosis of the lips, sweating, nausea, vomiting, and, in severe cases, rapid or slow heart rate, sudden shortness of breath, inability to lie down, low blood pressure, cold limbs, mottled skin, or even sudden death.

If these symptoms occur in a hospital, a heart attack is easily diagnosed. Hospitals have advanced equipment and diagnostic tools such as electrocardiograms, cardiac enzymes, coronary angiography, and myocardial perfusion imaging. However, if a heart attack occurs at home or elsewhere, without doctors or equipment (and even if one had the equipment, most people wouldn't know how to use it), you might only have a blood pressure monitor at most. So how can you tell if it's a heart attack?

You can only rely on the patient's symptoms. Self-awareness of symptoms is crucial, and the most typical symptom of a heart attack is the chest pain mentioned earlier.

There are two key locations where chest pain occurs: the precordial area and behind the sternum. The heart is about the size of the person's fist and is located in the center-left of the chest cavity. Roughly two-thirds of the heart is on the left side of the chest (the precordial area), while one-third is on the right side (behind the sternum).

Some of the most painful conditions in humans include:
1. Stones (such as gallstones or kidney stones)
2. Acute pancreatitis
3. Certain cancers (e.g., liver cancer, though the most painful cancer is pancreatic cancer, which is known as the "king of cancers" due to the extreme pain it causes).
Another very painful experience, though not a disease, is childbirth for women. Acute myocardial infarction is also one of the most painful conditions. I once treated a patient with a heart attack who was in such agony that he became restless and broke out in a cold sweat. It took two or three people to hold him down. His lips turned blue, and even his fingernails turned purple, with purple blotches appearing on his hands. I immediately administered diazepam to calm him down, which helped reduce his oxygen consumption and lowered the risk.

At this point, you may wonder: Why do heart attack patients experience chest pain?

The heart does not feel pain in response to mechanical stimuli. For example, if you stab the heart with a sharp object, it won't feel pain. However, the heart is extremely sensitive to a lack of oxygen. When the heart muscle becomes oxygen-deprived, it enters an anaerobic metabolic state, producing large amounts of acidic substances like lactic acid and pyruvic acid. The heart muscle is highly sensitive to these acids, which causes the pain.

That said, many causes of chest pain are not related to heart attacks.

Emergency Scene

There was a driver at our emergency center, Mr. Duan, who later transferred to a newspaper office. One morning, he came to the emergency center to see me. His face was pale, and he was clutching his chest, saying, "Dr. Jia, my chest hurts, and I feel short of breath." Mr. Duan was known for his sense of humor, so at first, I thought he was joking. Chest pain can be faked, but pale skin can't be.

Seeing how pale he was, I quickly had him lie down on a bench and asked a nurse to perform an electrocardiogram (ECG). It turned out to be a typical pattern of acute inferior wall myocardial infarction. While listening to his chest with a stethoscope, I noticed reduced breath sounds on the right side. After tapping on both sides of his chest, I found tympanic sounds on the right side and weakened vocal resonance. I asked him to take a deep breath, and he replied, "It hurts a lot when I breathe in." I then asked him to cough, and he said, "No, coughing makes it worse."

I told him, "It's not a heart attack. Go get a chest X-ray."

A little later, he came back with the X-ray and said, "Dr. Jia, I have a pneumothorax."

I laughed and said, "You're the one with a pneumothorax."

Sure enough, the X-ray confirmed a pneumothorax.
He asked, "What should I do?"

I told him, "Your lung compression is less than 30%, so there's no need for treatment."

I then asked him, "What did you do this morning?"
He said, "Nothing much... oh, I remember now! I slammed the car door a bit hard."

That could have been the cause. A few days later, when I saw Mr. Duan again, he had completely recovered.

What is a Pneumothorax?

A normal person's chest cavity is a sealed space under negative pressure. If air enters the chest cavity, the lung tissue will be compressed and unable to expand fully. If a chest X-ray shows less than 30% compression and there are no other serious symptoms, the situation isn't too serious, and no special treatment is needed. After some rest, it will heal naturally. This condition is called primary pneumothorax or idiopathic pneumothorax.

How can we distinguish between a heart attack and pneumothorax based on chest pain?

Generally, the onset of chest pain in pneumothorax is sudden, reaching its peak quickly. It's accompanied by shortness of breath, worsens with coughing or deep breaths, lasts for a shorter time, and is usually one-sided. If you tap on both sides of the chest, the sound will be different. Pneumothorax is more common in young adults, especially tall and thin men. On the other hand, chest pain caused by a heart attack is much more severe and typically occurs in people over 40 years old.

So, chest pain doesn't always mean a heart attack. Even if the ECG shows a typical heart attack pattern, it might not necessarily be a heart attack. In these situations, it's important for patients to trust their doctors, who will make a comprehensive assessment.

Pain is an unpleasant experience, but it's also a warning signal. Chest pain caused by a heart attack works the same way—it alerts us to a problem in the body. This way, we can call for emergency help and get to the hospital quickly, preventing tragedy.

Simple Differentiation Between Heart Attack and Pneumothorax

Heart Attack (Myocardial Infarction)	Pneumothorax
Chest pain often occurs behind the sternum or in the precordial area and can radiate to the left arm, back, or shoulder, often accompanied by symptoms such as chest tightness and shortness of breath.	The chest pain starts suddenly and rapidly reaches its peak, accompanied by shortness of breath. Coughing or deep breathing can exacerbate the pain.
The pain lasts longer, typically more than 30 minutes, and is very intense.	The pain lasts for a shorter duration and is usually confined to one side.
Commonly seen in individuals over 40 years of age.	Generally seen in younger adults, particularly tall and thin males.

Some symptoms, although not typical, can also be dangerous.

When acute myocardial infarction (AMI) presents with typical symptoms, it is usually not overlooked. However, atypical symptoms can easily be confused with other conditions, which often leads to insufficient attention. Many people may not even think to call for emergency assistance or seek medical care promptly. As a result, the condition can worsen and may even become life-threatening.

Acute myocardial infarction with atypical symptoms can be more frightening than when typical symptoms are present.

Symptom	Description
Throat Pain	Sudden throat pain without inflammation, especially accompanied by palpitations, chest tightness, sweating, etc. Often seen in those with high blood pressure, coronary heart disease, diabetes, or

Symptom	Description
	other conditions.
Abdominal Pain	Severe pain in the upper abdomen, soft stomach muscles, and tenderness without worsening upon pressure. Often accompanied by palpitations, nausea, vomiting, or cold sweats, particularly in those with a history of heart disease.
Toothache	Unexplained and persistent toothache without redness or swelling of the gums. Accompanied by palpitations, chest discomfort, nausea, vomiting, or facial pallor.
Other Symptoms	No chest pain but instead abdominal pain, accompanied by symptoms like nausea, vomiting, or pain in the head, neck, jaw, shoulders, or back. Unexplained fatigue, dizziness, or restlessness may also occur.

■ **Sore Throat**

Emergency Scene

A few years ago, a 50-year-old researcher called the head of the local clinic, complaining of a sore throat. The head replied, "Stay at home, I'll come over right away." When the head of the clinic arrived, he took the researcher's temperature—no fever, and the throat wasn't red or swollen, but the patient still felt a persistent sore throat. The head was puzzled and couldn't figure out the problem. Suddenly, he had a thought: could it be an atypical presentation of a heart condition? He immediately dialed the emergency number, 120. Around 11 p.m., we received the call to rescue the patient.

We performed an electrocardiogram (ECG) on the patient, and it turned out to be an acute anterior myocardial infarction. After emergency treatment, the patient requested to be transferred to the Beijing Emergency Center. The researcher's boss, upon hearing that his subordinate had suffered an acute myocardial infarction, rushed over and immediately agreed, "Don't worry about the costs; I'll cover them. Get to the emergency center right away." So, the patient was transferred to the Beijing Emergency Center, where he received interventional treatment.

On the day of his discharge, the patient specifically sought me out to express his gratitude, saying, "Thank you for saving my life!" I replied, "If you want to thank someone, don't thank me. Go thank the head of your clinic. If he had said, 'It's just a sore throat; everyone gets one. Let's talk about it in the morning,' you might not have made it until the next morning. Or if he had said, 'Your throat is sore, but it's not red, swollen, or feverish. Sore throats are usually due to inflammation; I'll prescribe some anti-inflammatory drugs and lozenges for you,' you might not have survived either. It was quite remarkable that the head could connect a sore throat to a potential heart attack; this isn't something that anti-inflammatory drugs could resolve."

The researcher laughed and said, "You're right, I

must thank him too!" I added, "And you should also thank your institute's director; otherwise, he wouldn't have covered your medical expenses." The researcher laughed heartily. Seeing his joy, I genuinely felt happy for him.

Generally speaking, the most common cause of a sore throat is inflammation, often due to a cold. In such cases, the throat may initially feel dry, like it's burning, and may swell up, with the pain radiating to the ears. In severe cases, fever, headaches, and body aches may occur.

However, if a sore throat suddenly develops, especially accompanied by palpitations, chest tightness, shortness of breath, or sweating, it should be considered as a potential atypical presentation of an acute myocardial infarction. This is particularly important if the patient has a history of high blood pressure, coronary heart disease, or diabetes. In such cases, call 120 and go to the hospital immediately.

■ Upper Abdominal Pain

Emergency Scene

Let me clarify right away: this is not a joke... One day, we received a dispatch, and the form said "upper abdominal pain." When we arrived at the patient's home, we found a man in his 40s lying sideways on the couch, looking restless, pale-faced, with lips turning blue and clothes soaked with sweat. I quickly approached, gently tapped his shoulder, and asked what was wrong. He struggled to open his eyes and weakly replied, "Stomach ache."

I asked his wife and son nearby. His wife said, "He's had this stomach pain for over an hour; it's really severe. Look, he's in so much pain that he's turned pale, struggling to breathe, and soaked in sweat! Please, get him to the hospital quickly!"

I felt the patient's abdomen—it was soft. Pressing on it didn't increase or reduce the pain.

Given the symptoms, it seemed likely that the issue was with his heart. I immediately instructed the nurse to perform an ECG. However, his son objected, "Why are you doing an ECG for stomach pain? Get him to the hospital now!" I explained that I was concerned the problem might be with the heart, not the stomach. The son got agitated, saying, "Heart problem? You just want to charge us more for unnecessary tests! Stop wasting time, get him to the hospital!"

Seeing the urgency, I insisted to the nurse, "Do it now!" I then turned to the family and said, "Let's do this: I'll waive the ECG fee if it's not a heart issue! I'll even waive the consultation and ambulance fees! How about that?" Without waiting for a response, the nurse quickly placed the electrodes, and I checked the patient's blood pressure—it was around 200 mmHg, with a pulse of about 30 beats per minute. I whispered to the nurse, "Inferior wall." The nurse understood, and after the ECG was performed, it confirmed acute inferior myocardial infarction with third-degree atrioventricular block. I immediately instructed the nurse to check the posterior wall and right ventricle since an acute inferior myocardial infarction often involves the posterior wall and right ventricle as well. The ECG results further confirmed extensive myocardial necrosis in the patient! His heart rate was 28 beats per minute—a life-threatening arrhythmia! This kind of cardiogenic shock, even with all-out resuscitation efforts, has a mortality rate of over 85%. Adding third-degree atrioventricular block made the situation extremely dire.

The family members turned pale with fear, and the patient's son fell to his knees, pleading through tears, "Doctor, I'm sorry for what I said earlier. Please, save my dad!" I helped him up and assured him that we would do everything we could to save him! We closely monitored the patient, continuously checking his blood pressure and heart rate, adjusting medication dosages accordingly. After half an hour, the patient became less agitated. His heart rate was around 60 beats per minute, and his blood pressure was 100/80 mmHg, meeting the criteria for transfer at that time (the transfer criteria have since been updated). We immediately transported him to the hospital for coronary angiography, and a stent was placed in the blocked coronary artery. The patient was incredibly fortunate—he was discharged safely after a few days, and everything turned out well in the end!

Not long ago, I saw a news story about a doctor suggesting an ECG for a patient with stomach pain, only to be beaten by the patient's family. In the midst of the fight, the patient had a heart attack... I couldn't help but joke to myself: honestly, I was also sweating a bit at that time— if the ECG had shown it wasn't a heart attack, I might have been the one kneeling…

I once shared this case on my social media, and a young doctor left a comment: "Why are you bragging? How could you know it was an inferior wall myocardial infarction before doing the ECG?" Clearly, this doctor lacked experience in such cases. I replied, "An inferior wall myocardial infarction is the most likely cause of upper abdominal pain and third-degree atrioventricular block. When I measured the blood pressure and heard a pulse of around 30 beats per minute, I suspected a fatal bradyarrhythmia—severe atrioventricular block. So, even before the ECG, I was already thinking it was an acute inferior myocardial infarction." This kind of diagnostic ability isn't boasting. Many skilled doctors at the Beijing Emergency Center possess such judgment; I'm merely an ordinary member of this exceptional group.

There are many causes of upper abdominal pain, such as issues with the stomach, duodenum, liver, gallbladder, or pancreas. However, sometimes heart problems can manifest as upper abdominal pain. Therefore, when elderly patients experience abdominal pain, especially those with a history of heart disease, and the pain is accompanied by symptoms like chest tightness, palpitations, sweating, cyanosis around the lips, and absence of tenderness in the pain area, the possibility of a heart condition should be considered. An ECG is crucial in such cases to avoid misdiagnosis.

■ Tooth Pain

For patients in critical condition, sudden death can be somewhat easier to accept. However, it's hard to imagine that something as minor as a toothache could be related to acute myocardial infarction or sudden death, even leading to death after a tooth extraction. Have you ever heard of such cases?

Deaths in dental clinics typically stem from two scenarios: oral cancer, which wouldn't cause sudden death, and facial injuries, which can be divided into two categories: massive bleeding leading to choking, or fractures of the maxilla causing suffocation due to downward displacement of the fracture segment pressing on the pharynx or airway.

If a patient dies immediately after a tooth extraction, it's almost certainly not due to a dental problem but rather an acute myocardial infarction! If a patient can't identify the exact tooth causing pain, and there is no redness, swelling, or tenderness of the teeth, but symptoms like chest tightness, breathlessness, chest discomfort, palpitations, sweating, and changes in facial appearance are present, it's important to consider whether an acute myocardial infarction is occurring.

During dental treatments, due to the patient's nervousness, adverse drug reactions, or the physical stress of the procedure, unexpected emergencies can occur, sometimes life-threatening ones. Therefore, before treating certain dental conditions, it's crucial to perform necessary physical examinations such as blood pressure measurement and ECG based on the patient's age, condition, psychological state, and medical history. This helps prevent or mitigate sudden incidents.

For this reason, I have been invited multiple times by the Beijing Oral Health Association and the National Medical Education Development Center to conduct seminars on "Managing Sudden Internal Emergencies in Dental Clinics" for dentists in Beijing and across the country. I've also recommended that dental clinics offer procedures under ECG monitoring, such as extractions, particularly for high-risk patients with hypertension or coronary heart disease.

The Beijing Dental Hospital at Xian Nong Tan took my advice early on and started offering ECG-monitored extractions. High-risk patients, such as those with hypertension and coronary artery disease, can now book appointments for these monitored procedures. I even recommended a retired doctor from the Beijing Emergency Center, known for his extensive experience in emergency care, to oversee this work at the Beijing Dental Hospital. Thanks to his efforts, many patients experiencing sudden complications during treatment have been stabilized.

■ Other Atypical Symptoms

There are many atypical symptoms of acute myocardial infarction. The following signs can all indicate a possible myocardial infarction and should be taken seriously: absence of chest pain, or only experiencing sensations like chest tightness, palpitations, and discomfort in the chest area; upper abdominal pain without chest pain, potentially accompanied by nausea and vomiting, which can easily be mistaken for acute abdominal conditions; pain in the jaw, neck, throat, teeth, shoulders, back, or arms without chest pain, which may be misdiagnosed as joint, bone, or soft tissue issues; and unexplained fainting, heart failure, or shock, which should all prompt consideration of a potential myocardial infarction.

Professor Chen Zaijia, former director of cardiology at Fuwai Hospital in Beijing, reported extremely rare cases where pain in areas like the head, lower limbs, and toes also manifested as atypical symptoms of myocardial infarction, making it difficult to connect to heart disease. However, if such pain is accompanied by symptoms like chest tightness, shortness of breath, palpitations, or sweating, it should still prompt suspicion of a myocardial infarction. In short, recognizing the signs of acute myocardial infarction, especially atypical ones, is crucial for timely diagnosis. Only by identifying it early can we prevent delays and potentially reduce instances of sudden death. Atypical symptoms are particularly dangerous because they are often overlooked.

People who experience a heart attack without chest pain usually fall into three groups: elderly individuals, women, and people with diabetes. These groups tend to have a lower sensitivity to pain, which increases their risk. The absence of chest pain is the most dangerous scenario. Therefore, these individuals and their families should remain vigilant. If any unusual symptoms occur, especially in elderly or diabetic patients, they should immediately stop any physical activity, lie down to rest, and calm themselves. Family members should closely monitor the patient's condition, and if symptoms persist or worsen, they should call 120 immediately and begin first aid. Never let the patient tough it out.

For women, more than half may not experience chest pain but may instead have unexplained symptoms like stomach pain, toothache, indigestion, sore throat, or pain in the shoulders and arms, which can last only a few minutes. If these symptoms occur, women should be extra cautious, particularly those with high blood pressure, diabetes, or a family history of heart attacks. They should consider the possibility of an acute myocardial infarction and seek medical attention as soon as possible.

Young People Are at Greater Risk from Heart Attacks

Many people have visited my blog to ask questions like, "Who is more likely to have a heart attack?" "Can heart attacks be prevented?" "Can young people have heart disease?" … It's clear that there's still a lot of misunderstanding about heart attacks.

So, who exactly is more prone to heart attacks, and how can they be prevented?

First, putting aside genetic factors, those who have unhealthy habits like staying up late or smoking are most likely to suffer from heart attacks. The news often reports cases where employees of foreign companies or programmers, due to high work stress and consecutive late nights, suffer sudden deaths. These so-called "death from overwork" cases are mostly caused by acute myocardial infarctions.

In the Asia-Pacific region, the top three risk factors for cardiovascular disease are hypertension, smoking, and high blood sugar. High-energy foods, as well as diets that are too salty or oily, are bad for the heart because they can cause a sudden rise in blood lipid levels, increasing blood viscosity, which can easily lead to heart attacks.

Medical research has found that people with abdominal obesity tend to have lower levels of "good cholesterol" in their blood, which increases the risk of heart disease. North Korea's former leaders, Kim Il-sung and Kim Jong-il, both had abdominal obesity. Even with doctors and caregivers always by their sides, they both eventually died from heart attacks.

Secondly, in terms of age, middle-aged and elderly people are the most susceptible to acute myocardial infarction. As people age, their metabolic rate decreases, the elasticity and flexibility of their blood vessels decrease, blood viscosity increases, and lipid metabolism disorders occur. These are all risk factors for coronary artery disease, of which heart attacks are a serious type. So, naturally, middle-aged and older adults are at higher risk. If they don't pay attention to their lifestyle habits, the chances of having a heart attack increase even more.

But if I were to ask, "Who is at greater risk from a heart attack, a 30-year-old or a 60-year-old?" Many people might immediately assume it's the 60-year-old. In reality, the 30-year-old is actually at greater risk. Why?

A person who experiences a heart attack at 60 may have already started developing coronary artery disease in their 30s, which means they might have developed a relatively complete "collateral circulation." By the time they reach 60, if a blood clot forms in their coronary artery, blocking blood flow, the collateral circulation can kick in, allowing blood to flow through alternative pathways, limiting the area of myocardial infarction. However, if a 30-year-old suddenly experiences a heart attack, their coronary artery's collateral circulation might not have had time to develop. So, if a blood clot forms, the situation is far more dangerous.

So, what is collateral circulation? Let me give you an example.

The blood vessels in the body are like the roads in Beijing. The major arteries are like the main roads, such as Chang'an Avenue or Ping'an Avenue, while the collateral circulation represents smaller alleyways. When Chang'an Avenue is blocked, a smart driver can take the alleys and still reach their destination. Our body has a similar self-regulating mechanism—if a blockage occurs in one area, over time, it can develop collateral circulation to bypass the blockage.

Emergency Scene

This reminds me of an incident where I helped save the life of a 19-year-old Air Force cadet.

One morning around 7 a.m., at the Nanyuan Airport of the Air Force, a 19-year-old cadet suddenly felt chest discomfort while doing laundry. His fellow cadets quickly took him to the airport hospital on a bicycle. Just as he entered the hospital doors, he collapsed to the ground and lost consciousness. It was around 7:50 a.m., just as the doctors and nurses were starting their shifts, so they immediately moved him to the emergency room for resuscitation. Meanwhile, the airport hospital's doctors made emergency calls for assistance to the Air Force General Hospital, the nearby 711 Hospital of the Aerospace Ministry, and the Beijing Emergency Center.

We learned that the hospital was performing CPR on the patient and rushed to the Nanyuan Airport Hospital. As soon as we got out of the car, a group of military personnel surrounded us, and someone introduced me to a political commissar. The commissar said, "Now that the emergency team is here, I'm relieved." I replied, "Don't be too optimistic just yet; I haven't seen the patient."

Entering the emergency room, I found over 10 doctors and nurses working intensely. The patient had no spontaneous heartbeat or respiration. The anesthetist from the 711 Hospital, who had arrived first, had already intubated the patient and was performing manual ventilation with an oxygen bag. Another doctor from the airport hospital was doing external cardiac compressions, with an IV line in place and ECG monitoring connected. A doctor from the Air Force General Hospital had also arrived before me.

I quickly assessed the medication being administered. Suddenly, I noticed rhythmic activity on the ECG monitor and instructed the doctor performing chest compressions, "Stop, stop, let me check." Sure enough, the monitor showed "ventricular tachycardia," which was a positive sign, but not yet a cause for optimism, as it could easily deteriorate into "ventricular fibrillation." We needed to correct it to a "sinus rhythm" immediately.

The doctor from the Air Force General Hospital immediately called for "lidocaine," while I simultaneously said, "synchronized cardioversion!" Grabbing the two paddles from the defibrillator, I got ready. Our emergency nurse charged the defibrillator and applied conductive gel to the paddles. Within seconds, we were ready. I placed the paddles on the patient's chest and commanded, "Shock!" The defibrillator's screen displayed "sinus rhythm," and everyone in the room breathed a sigh of relief. At that moment, the lidocaine hadn't even been administered yet. The patient soon began to breathe spontaneously, with a blood pressure reading of 120/80 mmHg. It was a moment of pure relief!

Suddenly, the patient began to have seizures, caused by brain swelling due to hypoxia. I quickly asked, "Has he been given diuretics?" A doctor replied, "Yes, we've given 500 ml of mannitol."

I said, "Draw 20 mg of diazepam for IV injection."

The Air Force General Hospital doctor responded, "10 mg!" So, the nurse administered 10 mg of diazepam, but the patient continued to seize. Less than a minute later, the seizures stopped but then resumed within another minute.

I insisted again, "Draw 20 mg of diazepam for IV injection." The doctor from the Air Force General

Hospital still didn't follow my suggestion. This back-and-forth happened two or three times, and a total of 30 mg of diazepam was administered, but the patient continued to seize, with brief pauses followed by more seizures.

The Air Force General Hospital doctor asked, "Is there any other option?"

I replied, "You didn't follow my advice. I said to draw 20 mg, not to inject it all at once. Sometimes, just 1 vial could stop the seizures; other times, it might take a bit more. The key is to stop injecting as soon as the seizures stop. This way, you can control the seizures effectively while avoiding cumulative toxicity from repeated dosing. By administering it your way, not only has the total amount of medication increased beyond what I suggested, but the effectiveness is also poorer." He remained silent.

Later, the patient was still seizing, and the Air Force General Hospital doctor asked me again, "Is there any other way?"

I said, "Now, the patient's heartbeat, respiration,

blood pressure, and pulse are stable. There are no arrhythmias, heart failure, or shock. He can be transported to the hospital while receiving continuous care during the transfer." Afterward, we loaded the patient into the Air Force General Hospital's vehicle.

The next afternoon, I called the Nanyuan Airport Hospital to check on the patient's condition. They were thrilled to tell me, "The patient has regained consciousness without any lasting complications. We just got back from the hospital—he's already able to eat watermelon."

Therefore, I want to remind young people not to think that heart attacks are far from them or to ignore physical discomfort. In reality, heart attacks are occurring at younger ages, and they are no longer just a concern for middle-aged and older adults.

Since heart attacks can happen to anyone, prevention is crucial. The most economical and effective way to prevent heart attacks is through exercise. However, exercise should be done correctly, so what's the best approach?

For healthy young people, various aerobic exercises are great options. But for middle-aged and older individuals, who might have limitations in their legs and knees, what should they do? Walking or swimming are good choices, with swimming being one of the best forms of exercise. Water's buoyancy helps relax the joints and spine, making it especially suitable for older adults with joint issues.

One more point to emphasize: consistency is key in exercise. Sporadic efforts won't do much good.

Learning New Emergency Skills: The "357" Exercise Rule

The "3" stands for 30 minutes or 3 kilometers. It means engaging in exercises like brisk walking or jogging for 30 minutes daily or covering a distance of 3 kilometers. It's both economical and effective.

The "5" means exercising at least 5 days a week.

The "7" refers to maintaining an optimal heart rate during exercise, calculated as "170 minus your age." For example, if I am 60 years old,then 170-60=110, so my ideal exercise heart rate is around 110 beats per minute.

Four Steps for Heart Attack First Aid

Learn New First Aid Skills Together

Pre-hospital Emergency Measures for Acute Myocardial Infarction

Step 1: Help the patient calm down and rest quietly, avoiding any further stress.

Step 2: Help the patient find a comfortable position.
- If the patient is experiencing difficulty breathing, assist them into a sitting position with their legs hanging down. Make sure the position is as comfortable as possible.
- If the patient's blood pressure drops, or if they go into shock, lay them flat, remove any pillows, keep them warm, and prevent choking due to vomiting.
- If difficulty breathing, low blood pressure, and shock occur simultaneously, place the patient in

a semi-reclining position and adjust the angle as needed.

Step 3: If oxygen is available, have the patient use it at a flow rate of 3-5 liters per minute. Depending on the situation, have the patient chew 100-300 mg of aspirin.

Step 4: Call emergency services (120) and be ready to perform CPR at any time.

Step 1: Help the Patient Rest and Avoid Stress

If the patient experiences chest pain during physical activity, have them stop immediately. If they are emotionally agitated, try to calm them down. A common scene in TV dramas is an elderly father getting upset and clutching his chest suddenly. This is not a fictional scenario; heart attacks are often related to emotions. In such moments, no matter the conflict, avoid provoking them further. A simple "It's my fault, please don't be upset" can calm the situation.

Step 2: Help the Patient Find a Comfortable Position

What is a comfortable position? It's based on how the patient feels—lying down or sitting.
- If the patient has difficulty breathing, it may indicate acute left heart failure. Help them sit up with their legs hanging down, making the position as comfortable as possible. This can reduce pressure on the lungs from abdominal organs, helping maintain lung ventilation, and more importantly, reduce the volume of blood returning to the heart due to gravity, thus lowering the heart's workload.
- If the patient's blood pressure drops or they go into shock, lay them flat, even removing pillows, and keep them warm. Be cautious to prevent choking if they vomit.
- If both acute left heart failure and shock occur together, it becomes particularly challenging. Lying flat can worsen breathing difficulty, while sitting up can decrease blood flow to the brain, potentially causing unconsciousness. The best approach is to place the patient in a semi-reclining position and adjust as needed, though it

may still be uncomfortable.

Step 3: Provide Oxygen and Medication

If there is an oxygen cylinder at home, administer oxygen to the patient at a rate of 3-5 liters per minute. This has a dual function of providing medical assistance and psychological comfort, as it can increase oxygen supply to the heart and alleviate symptoms. If oxygen is not available, focus on medication. It's advisable for households, especially those with elderly members, to keep emergency medications like nitroglycerin and aspirin, which can be crucial in critical moments.

Nitroglycerin is a common medication for heart disease patients. Place one tablet (0.5 mg) under the patient's tongue; it takes effect in 1-3 minutes and can be repeated after 10 minutes, but no more than three tablets in total.

It is important to note that if possible, measure the patient's blood pressure before using nitroglycerin, as acute myocardial infarction often comes with low blood pressure or even shock. Using nitroglycerin in such cases can cause further drops in blood pressure, which may be life-threatening. Make sure blood pressure stays within a safe range during use. Specifically, if a patient's usual blood pressure is 120 mmHg and rises to 140 mmHg during an episode, using nitroglycerin is generally safe. However, if their usual blood pressure is 120 mmHg but drops to 100 mmHg during an episode, nitroglycerin should be avoided, as it could worsen the condition. If the patient experiences dizziness, palpitations, or pale skin after taking the medication, measure their blood pressure immediately, stop the medication if it is low, and have the patient lie down.

Additionally, besides low blood pressure, patients with a fast or slow heart rate, acute inferior myocardial infarction, acute right ventricular myocardial infarction, or those who have taken Viagra in the past 24-48 hours should not use nitroglycerin.

A reminder: Nitroglycerin should be stored in a dark, airtight container, carried with the patient but not "on their person" because body heat can affect its potency and reduce its shelf life.

After following these steps, if the patient's chest pain quickly subsides, it is generally considered "angina." If the pain does not subside, or even worsens, it might indicate acute myocardial infarction. If a heart attack is strongly suspected, it is not advisable to use nitroglycerin. Nitroglycerin does not treat acute myocardial infarction and may even worsen the condition in some cases. At this point, 100-300 mg of aspirin may be chewed, as it has anticoagulant properties that can prevent the enlargement of blood clots, the formation of new clots, and limit the extent of heart muscle damage. It's also important to consider other possible causes of chest pain besides coronary artery disease, such as expired medications. If the patient is allergic to aspirin or has a history of aortic dissection, gastrointestinal bleeding, or brain hemorrhage, they should not take aspirin.

Some heart patients may use a medication called "Suxiao Jiuxin Wan" (Cardiotonic Pills). However, despite the name "fast-acting," its efficacy is not comparable to that of nitroglycerin or aspirin.

In situations where it is unclear whether to use nitroglycerin or aspirin, the patient should immediately call 120 and let emergency personnel determine the appropriate medication. Acute myocardial infarction patients should never attempt to go to the hospital on their own; they must call 120 and let doctors perform necessary treatment before deciding when to transfer them to the hospital.

Step 4: Call 120 and Be Ready for CPR

As we know, acute myocardial infarction is a highly dangerous condition with a high risk of sudden death, and the patient could experience cardiac arrest at any time. It is essential to be prepared to perform CPR on the spot.

If someone in the household experiences an acute myocardial infarction, in addition to chewing aspirin and calling 120 immediately, it is crucial to be ready to perform CPR if needed.

A reminder: When dealing with an acute myocardial infarction patient, those nearby (such as family members) should avoid moving the patient casually. Moving a heart attack patient can increase oxygen consumption by the heart, placing extra stress on it and potentially enlarging the infarct area, worsening the condition, and triggering sudden death—what could be a well-intentioned mistake. Typically, emergency doctors will stabilize the patient's condition before transporting them, ensuring their condition is suitable for transfer before taking them to the hospital for further examination and treatment, thus preventing complications and deterioration.

Pre-hospital emergency care is crucial, but timely hospitalization is just as essential.

Emergency Scene

Once, I arrived at a patient's residence, where a taxi was parked outside. The taxi driver approached me and said, "Doctor, there's a patient here who wanted to take my taxi. When they came out, I could tell right away that it looked like a heart attack—they were sweating profusely, with a bluish tint on their lips. It looked serious, so I didn't dare take them. Instead, I helped them sit on the steps and called 120 for them."

When I entered the patient's home and conducted an ECG, it turned out to be acute myocardial infarction. After I finished stabilizing the patient and came back outside, the taxi driver was still there. I informed him about the patient's condition, and he even helped us lift the patient into the ambulance. Together with the family, I thanked him. He smiled proudly, "No problem, no problem! It's my duty!" He then whispered to me, "A while back, I had a similar case, but that person died of a heart attack in my taxi."

This taxi driver was well-informed, and I've encountered such cases four or five times. We should truly appreciate these drivers—without their caution, patients who attempt to go directly to the hospital in a taxi might die on the way.

However, not everyone has the awareness of this taxi driver. Some do not realize that before transporting a heart attack patient to the hospital, essential on-site emergency care is necessary. Timely admission and observation in a hospital is absolutely crucial.

I also recall a time when I treated Mr. Qian Jiaxiang, a renowned figure in Chinese sports. He was once the Vice Chairman of the China Volleyball Association and Chairman of the Asian Volleyball Confederation's Competition

Committee. In the 1940s, he was a volleyball star and even coached Yuan Weimin.

On the night of February 4, 1989, at around 1 a.m., Mr. Qian Jiaxiang suddenly experienced chest pain without other accompanying symptoms. When I arrived at his home, I immediately performed an ECG, which appeared mostly normal, showing no signs of "acute myocardial infarction" or "arrhythmia." After a thorough examination, I administered intravenous nitroglycerin, and the chest pain subsided within a few minutes. I said, "You still need to go to the hospital, but now you can go." Mr. Qian got up to put on his clothes, but I stopped him, saying, "You can't move on your own; you need to be carried."

The nurse present gave me a puzzled look, but after years of working together, I understood what she meant: "The ECG is normal, the chest pain is gone—why the need to carry him?" Although the ECG was normal and his symptoms had disappeared, my professional intuition, honed over many years, told me that it wasn't just angina, but likely an acute myocardial infarction. If I didn't consider the possibility of a heart attack, I would have let him walk down the stairs himself, or perhaps not even required him to go to the hospital at all. But since I suspected this life-threatening condition, I couldn't let him walk; he needed to be carried out on a stretcher. Why? If a heart attack patient moves around, it increases their myocardial oxygen consumption, adding stress to the heart. Even minor activities, like climbing stairs, can increase heart rate, further increasing the heart's oxygen demand. This can be extremely dangerous, potentially leading to sudden death.

Mr. Qian's wife, a former member of the first generation of China's national women's volleyball team and a native of Shanghai, didn't want to inconvenience others, so she was reluctant to seek help. Despite my repeated explanations of the risks, she insisted that they shouldn't trouble anyone, and no one was called. Meanwhile, there were only three of us present, and we couldn't carry the tall Mr. Qian Jiaxiang down the stairs ourselves.

After more than 10 minutes, I performed another

ECG, and it confirmed my earlier intuition. The ECG displayed classic signs of an "acute extensive anterior myocardial infarction." The patient subsequently experienced repeated severe and complex life-threatening arrhythmias, but fortunately, each time, we managed to stabilize him with timely medication. I continued to monitor his heart rhythm, measuring his blood pressure frequently and performing an ECG every 20-30 minutes to observe any changes in his condition.

Throughout the night, I continuously informed the family about his condition and stressed the urgency of hospital admission. I repeatedly urged Mrs. Qian to find help to carry Mr. Qian downstairs to the ambulance, but she remained adamant. In fact, since they lived in the residential complex of the National Sports Commission, finding a few people to help would have been easy. Mr. Qian Jiaxiang remained conscious throughout and even joked and chatted with me about Beijing opera, though I didn't have the heart to engage in conversation. It wasn't until after 7 a.m. that Mrs. Qian finally called for help. Before transporting the patient to the ambulance, I conducted a thorough check to ensure he met the conditions for transfer. Unknowingly, more than six hours had passed, and we had all spent a sleepless night together.

Those six hours were truly nerve-wracking and felt like an eternity. Although I couldn't rush or express frustration, I was relieved when Mrs. Qian finally sought help. About 10 minutes later, we safely transported Mr. Qian to the Beijing Emergency Center. Once we arrived, I handed the patient over to the emergency department doctors. Since I was on the emergency shift, it was time for me to go home, but knowing how serious his condition was, I decided to stay and see how the rescue efforts would proceed. As expected, Mr. Qian continued to experience various severe, complex, life-threatening arrhythmias, and his blood pressure became undetectable. The Emergency Center quickly called in renowned experts like Professor Song Youcheng from Beijing Fuwai Hospital, Professor Shen Luhua from Beijing Friendship Hospital, and another specialist from People's Hospital. These top experts from four major hospitals collaborated in a high-level rescue effort.

The Director of the National Sports Commission, Yuan Weimin, Training Bureau Director Wu Shouzhang, and Volleyball Department Director Zhou Xiaolan also rushed to the Emergency Center, staying by Mr. Qian Jiaxiang's side.

Despite the experts' best efforts, they were ultimately unable to save Mr. Qian Jiaxiang, who passed away at the age of 63. After his passing, *Sports News* and *New Sports* magazines both reported the event accurately. At the scene of Mr. Qian's initial rescue, only four people were present—Mr. Qian, his wife, myself, and a nurse. With the patient gone, the reporters did not interview the nurse or me, so it was only Mrs. Qian who could provide the details of what happened.

We often encounter situations where family members try to help a patient with acute myocardial infarction out of their home, only for the patient to suddenly collapse and die just outside the door. It's truly tragic.

Therefore, "on-site emergency care" is one of the principles for managing acute myocardial infarction. But this principle can be misunderstood. When we say "don't move," it means the patient should lie still and avoid activity during a heart attack, not that others shouldn't "move" the patient. In reality, once a myocardial infarction occurs and the patient's condition stabilizes, they should be transported to a hospital with advanced care as soon as possible. The sooner they receive treatment, the higher the chances of a successful outcome, and the better the recovery. On the other hand, the longer the delay, the greater the area of myocardial damage, the more challenging the treatment, and the less effective the recovery. If blood flow is restored within 2 hours of a heart attack, most of the heart muscle can recover. For every additional hour of delay, the mortality rate increases by 10%. Ideally, the patient should reach the hospital within 2 hours of symptom onset.

Of course, while this sounds straightforward,

during actual rescue situations, we may encounter various challenges and must adapt to the circumstances.

Please Give Doctors More Trust and Understanding at Critical Times

Treating patients and saving lives is our duty as doctors. Some people refer to us as "angels in white," but we certainly don't dare to take such a title. Others treat us like "living deities," believing that as long as we are on the scene, no matter how severe the patient's condition, we will always be able to save them. But that is far from reality. Sometimes, even if we make every effort in the rescue, following every step correctly, the result may still be unsuccessful. This outcome is often directly related to the severity of the patient's condition, especially for patients with acute myocardial infarction. When it reaches the point where blood pressure is undetectable, the chances of a successful rescue are truly very low.

Emergency Scene

1.

There was a time when one of my colleagues went to rescue a patient. As soon as he walked in, he realized the patient's condition was extremely serious—acute myocardial infarction, with no detectable blood pressure. When he informed the family about the severity, they became anxious and said, "Hurry, take him to the hospital!"

But my colleague insisted on staying put: "No, the patient's condition is too critical; moving him would be even more dangerous! We need to do some initial treatment here before going!"

After much back and forth, he finally managed to persuade the family, and he began emergency care. But emergency care doesn't guarantee that the patient will be saved. In the end, despite his efforts, the patient did not survive. The family was furious and kept accusing him: "I told you to go, but you refused. You delayed it, and now he's dead!"

That day, luck was not on his side. Later, he encountered another acute myocardial infarction patient, again in a very severe state with no blood pressure. The family again insisted, "He's in such a critical state; hurry to the hospital." My colleague again explained the principle of "on-site emergency care," just like before.

This time, the family said, "You're just afraid of taking responsibility, right? I'll write a note, saying we take full responsibility for the consequences if we go straight to the hospital without treatment. Now will you feel reassured?"

Seeing the note and thinking about the previous incident, my colleague thought, "Fine, if you insist, let's go!" So they left. Not long after getting into the vehicle, the patient stopped breathing and his heart stopped beating. Despite trying CPR, he couldn't be resuscitated. At this point, the family turned on him again: "Doctor, aren't heart patients supposed to avoid being moved? Don't you know that?"

My colleague replied, "Of course I know."

"Then why did you move him?" the family blamed him again.

"Wasn't it you who insisted on moving him? Didn't you write this note?" He held up the note, trembling with anger.

"Are you the doctor, or am I? I don't know better, but don't you? If you know better, why did you listen to me when I said to move?"

In the end, it was still seen as his fault. That day, my colleague was extremely upset, and I truly felt sorry for him. We understand the family's emotions; it's one thing for them to misunderstand us, but it's another when it results in the loss of a loved one's life.

2.

In our department, there is a Dr. Liang, who is about ten years older than me. When he was in his fifties, he once went to rescue a patient with acute myocardial infarction. When he arrived, the patient's condition wasn't particularly critical—they weren't in severe pain and were relatively calm. Dr. Liang performed an ECG and found that it was an acute anterior myocardial infarction with ventricular tachycardia, which meant that cardiac arrest was imminent. He immediately administered lidocaine to treat the ventricular tachycardia. However, despite the medication, the patient soon went into ventricular fibrillation—a fatal arrhythmia—and their heart stopped. Dr. Liang quickly began CPR, but it was unsuccessful, and the patient could not be saved.

Dr. Liang was alone at the scene, performing most of the procedures himself, and it was incredibly hectic. Readers, take note: the scene of a medical rescue is chaotic, especially when only one doctor is present. However, we may be busy, but we are not panicked. Dr. Liang's administration of medication and CPR were completely correct—any doctor in any hospital would have handled the situation the same way. But no one can guarantee that a rescue will always be successful. Unfortunately, many times, the patients and their families don't understand this, nor do they care.

At the time, the patient's son walked over and

slapped Dr. Liang across the face, hurling insults, saying, "When you arrived, my dad could still talk, but after you gave him the medication, he died. It was you who killed him, wasn't it?"

Dr. Liang felt utterly crushed at that moment. He had done nothing wrong, yet was misunderstood by the family, and at his age, he was struck by a young man. The patient's son was extremely emotional and could not listen to any explanation from the doctor.

3.

As emergency doctors, we often face physical assaults. Speaking of myself, I've been slapped several times, and I've had to replace multiple pairs of glasses! You might say, "Why do people keep hitting you? Maybe you deserved it!" That would be quite unfair!

Take one of my experiences: there have been many times when, as soon as I got out of the ambulance, a family member would grab me by the collar and yell, "Where the hell have you been?!" Traffic jams! The roads are always packed, and many drivers block the emergency lane. We don't have wings—we can't fly over them!

On another occasion, I rushed to Beijing University of Technology to save a patient. As soon as I got into the yard, I saw the patient lying on the ground without a pulse or breathing. I immediately knelt down to start CPR. Suddenly, a young man came running towards me with a kitchen knife in his hand, shouting furiously, "If you don't save my dad today, I'll kill you!"

What kind of logic is that?

It's not like I caused his father's condition—why threaten me? You might think I'm exaggerating, but situations like these are all too common for us. Many of our colleagues at the emergency center have been assaulted—some have been left with black eyes, head injuries, broken noses, or even broken legs. Who can we turn to for sympathy?

Doctors at our emergency center have

encountered situations like those described above many times, but there's nothing we can do. We understand the family's emotions—when a loved one is seriously ill or passes away, it's natural to be upset. We doctors can only bear the burden quietly.

Clinical Coronary Disease mentions some very rare atypical symptoms of myocardial infarction, such as headaches, pain in both lower limbs, or pain in the toes. These symptoms don't usually seem related to heart disease, but there is indeed an internal connection, even though it's hard to explain this relationship to the average person. As a result, we emergency doctors often face various challenges in our work. For example, if you complain of chest pain and I perform an ECG, no one questions it. If you have back pain and I do an ECG, that's understandable too. But if you have a headache and I run an ECG, you might raise an eyebrow. And if you have pain in your toes and I suggest an ECG, you might even think I'm just trying to run up the bill, right?

So, I'd like to tell the readers that no matter what,

doctors will always do their best to treat patients. However, medicine is not omnipotent, and doctors are not miracle workers who can bring people back from the brink of death. I hope that after reading this book, you not only gain some knowledge that can help in emergencies but also remember this: give doctors more understanding and trust, especially at critical moments. This is meaningful not just for the patients and their families, but also for us doctors.

Chapter 3: Acute Cerebrovascular Diseases: Distinguishing Symptoms Before Emergency Care

"Better a Heart Attack than a Stroke"—The Dangers of Acute Cerebrovascular Diseases

In the previous chapter, we discussed the dangers of heart attacks, and I believe everyone now has a better understanding of them. However, many people, myself included, would rather suffer from an acute heart attack than an acute cerebrovascular disease. Why is that?

Acute cerebrovascular diseases include hemorrhagic cerebrovascular diseases (such as cerebral hemorrhage) and ischemic cerebrovascular diseases (such as cerebral infarction and cerebral embolism). Hemorrhagic cerebrovascular disease refers to non-traumatic bleeding caused by the rupture of blood vessels within the brain tissue, accounting for 20% to 30% of all cerebrovascular diseases, with a mortality rate of 30% to 40% in the acute phase. Ischemic cerebrovascular disease occurs when a blood clot forms in the brain's arteries or an embolus from another part of the body travels through the bloodstream to the brain, blocking blood and oxygen supply to the affected brain tissue, resulting in tissue necrosis.

Acute cerebrovascular diseases have the characteristics of "Four Highs and One Low." The "Four Highs" are high incidence, high recurrence rate, high disability rate, and high mortality, while the "One Low" is the low cure rate.

Once someone suffers from an acute cerebrovascular disease, the outcome is often either death or disability. Even if they survive, they may be left with varying degrees of sequelae. The most severe outcome is becoming a "vegetative state," where the patient has only breathing and heartbeat, but no awareness, thought, emotions, language, or voluntary actions—essentially a "social death." Even if they are not in a vegetative state, their quality of life is significantly compromised.

If someone has an acute heart attack, most survivors can regain independence in daily activities and even return to work. Cerebrovascular disease is different. Although its sudden death rate is not as high as that of a heart attack, its cure rate is much lower, and patients often suffer from various sequelae. A large amount of data shows that among survivors of cerebrovascular disease, 50% to 80% are left with varying degrees of disability, such as hemiplegia, slurred speech, joint stiffness, cognitive decline, or dementia. About three-quarters of these patients lose their ability to work, and two-thirds require assistance with daily living. Furthermore, the suffering of patients is only one aspect of the burden of cerebrovascular disease; it also places a heavy burden on their families—financially, physically, and psychologically. No wonder there's a saying, "One stroke, the whole family breaks down."

While cerebrovascular disease affects the blood vessels, its most severe impact is on brain function. Many times, patients cannot fully recover.

In addition to its destructive nature, cerebrovascular disease is especially dangerous due to its high incidence. I have read a report that states that 1.5 to 2 million people in China suffer from cerebrovascular diseases each year. Moreover, as the population with "Three Highs" (high blood pressure, high blood sugar, and high cholesterol) increases, the number of cerebrovascular patients is growing rapidly at an annual rate of 8.7%, which is double the rate in the United States. The mortality rate of cerebrovascular disease in China is 4 to 6 times that of myocardial infarction, and the economic burden it brings is 10 times greater. Furthermore, the mortality rate from cerebrovascular diseases, mainly cerebral infarction and cerebral hemorrhage, accounts for 24.4% of all causes of death. What does this mean? It means that out of every four people who die, roughly one dies from cerebrovascular disease. Currently, the mortality rate from cerebrovascular disease in China is 116 per 100,000 people, making it the second leading cause of death.

In addition, cerebrovascular disease has many complications, such as weakened immune function, pneumonia, urinary tract infections, and bedsores.

It is particularly important to note that like heart attacks, cerebrovascular disease is increasingly affecting younger individuals. I have seen many cases of stroke in people in their 30s. Among those under 45, the incidence of cerebrovascular disease has nearly doubled compared to 10 years ago. This should be a cause for concern.

Given the many dangers of cerebrovascular disease, does this mean that there is no hope if someone suffers from it? Although the cure rate is low, there are still measures that can be taken—early and aggressive treatment is key. For patients with cerebrovascular disease, time is not only a matter of life but also a guarantee of quality of life.

"Smile, Raise, Speak": Recognize the Signs and Call 120 Immediately

As mentioned earlier, cerebrovascular diseases can be classified into hemorrhagic (e.g., cerebral hemorrhage) and ischemic (e.g., cerebral thrombosis) types. Although these two types are fundamentally different—one involves bleeding and the other, lack of blood flow—their symptoms are very similar. The most common symptoms in patients are sensory and motor disturbances in one side of the body.

How to Recognize a Cerebrovascular Episode?

If a patient exhibits any of the following symptoms, it may indicate the onset of a cerebrovascular event, and you don't need to worry about determining the exact type:

1. Headache or dizziness;

2. Nausea or vomiting (especially projectile vomiting), or drooling;

3. Weakness or even paralysis on one side of the body;

4. Slurred speech or complete inability to speak;

5. Incontinence of urine or stool;

6. Various levels of consciousness impairment, such as drowsiness, confusion, or even deep coma.

If you cannot determine the symptoms precisely, I can teach you a simple method to identify the onset of a cerebrovascular episode. Ask the patient to perform three actions: smile, raise their hands, and say their name and address. If the patient is unable to do any of these three actions, it is likely a cerebrovascular event—call 120 for emergency services immediately while beginning first aid measures.

Emergency Scene

One time, I received a phone call: "Mr. Jia, a few days ago, I attended your emergency first aid class, and I ended up using what I learned. One of my neighbors, who is in his 50s, usually gets up around six or seven in the morning. But that day, even after 8 o'clock, he still hadn't gotten out of bed. His wife called him for breakfast several times, but he didn't respond. She then went over to him and called again, but he still didn't move. Realizing something was wrong, she quickly called me over. As soon as I saw him, I remembered what you taught us about acute cerebrovascular diseases. I followed the method you taught us to determine that it might be a stroke. Since he was lying on his back and appeared nauseated as if he was about to vomit, I quickly turned him into the 'recovery position.' As soon as I turned him over, he vomited. Later, I called 120 for him. At the hospital, a CT scan confirmed it was a cerebral thrombosis. Looking back, I realize how frightening it could have been—if I hadn't followed your advice and turned him to the 'recovery position,' he might have suffocated."

Patients with acute cerebrovascular disease are highly prone to falling into a coma, usually due to a lack of oxygen in the brain. Hypoxia in the brain is also a major reason why many patients with cerebrovascular disease have poor recovery outcomes or suffer from severe long-term complications.

Coma is a typical symptom of patients with cerebral hemorrhage.

What is a coma? Simply put, it is a state in which the person cannot be awakened no matter how much you try, but they still have breathing and a heartbeat. In a coma, a person loses awareness and does not respond to external stimuli. For example, if you pinch a sleeping person hard, the pain will wake them up. But for someone in a coma, even a strong pinch will elicit no response.

Coma patients may not show significant changes in facial color, or they might have a flushed complexion, and their pulse can still be strong, with a "thumping" beat, and their blood pressure might even be high. A coma can occur gradually as consciousness is lost, or it can happen suddenly, with the patient becoming completely unresponsive.

Many people often confuse coma, syncope (fainting), and shock, not understanding the differences between them.

At the emergency center, we often receive calls saying that a patient is in shock. We rush to the scene with the ambulance, only to find everyone standing around. We ask where the patient is, and someone points, "Over there!" We turn and see the patient standing perfectly fine. I ask, "Wasn't this person in shock? How are they standing now?" And they reply, "They were in shock earlier, but they're better now." It's both amusing and frustrating. Similarly, we receive many calls about "comatose" patients.

In reality, those who are able to stand up afterward are not in a coma or shock; they've simply experienced syncope.

We often see such scenes in TV dramas: an elderly woman gets into an argument and suddenly faints, with people around her frantically trying to wake her up, shaking her until she regains consciousness. This is a classic example of syncope. The patient can be woken up quickly or gradually regain consciousness over time. After fainting, they are able to speak clearly, move their limbs, and have normal heart rate and blood pressure. In most cases, this is simple syncope and is not serious.

Syncope is a transient loss of consciousness due to a temporary reduction in blood flow to the brain, often caused by various factors. More than 90% of syncope cases are due to transient cerebral hypoperfusion. Syncope usually has a trigger, such as excessive fatigue, hunger, prolonged standing, or emotional stress.

Shock, on the other hand, is a state in which the effective circulating blood volume suddenly drops due to various causes, leading to insufficient microcirculatory perfusion, which in turn causes tissue hypoxia, metabolic disturbances, and dysfunction of multiple organs.

What situations can cause a person to go into shock? The most common cause is severe bleeding. This is easy to understand—when too much blood is lost, the volume in the body decreases, and eventually there is not enough, leading to shock. Additionally, severe sweating, diarrhea, or vomiting can cause a significant loss of bodily fluids. While the red blood cells, white blood cells, platelets, and other components of the blood do not decrease, the loss of fluids leads to reduced blood volume, which can also cause shock.

Shock has two major characteristic manifestations: one is a significant drop in the patient's blood pressure, often to the point where it can't be measured, and their pulse becomes undetectable; the other is peripheral circulatory disturbances, such as cold hands and feet, pale complexion, bluish lips, and altered consciousness. At the onset of shock, the person's consciousness may remain relatively clear, but as blood flow to the brain continues to decrease, their awareness becomes increasingly impaired, leading to drowsiness and eventually loss of consciousness.

Of course, if you're unable to distinguish between shock, coma, and syncope, there's no need to panic. If you notice that the patient's condition is deteriorating, in addition to administering any necessary first aid measures, call 120 immediately, clearly describe the patient's condition, and wait for the doctor to arrive and provide further assistance.

Comparison table of shock, coma and syncope

Condition	Specific Symptoms of the Patient	Urgency Level
Shock	Pale complexion, irritability, restlessness, slow reflexes, pale face, clammy skin (cold to the touch), weak breathing, faint pulse (even	★★★★★

Condition	Specific Symptoms of the Patient	Urgency Level
	undetectable), blood pressure drops to undetectable levels, no urine or bowel movements, consciousness is unclear or even comatose.	
Coma	Facial color is unchanged or flushed, patient is unresponsive to calls but has breathing and a heartbeat; the loss of consciousness may be sudden or gradual.	★★★★
Syncope	Usually caused by overexertion, emotional stress, or similar factors; patients may have symptoms like pale complexion, shallow breathing, sweating, dilated pupils, limb muscle relaxation, and cold extremities. Some may lose consciousness, but	★★★

Condition	Specific Symptoms of the Patient	Urgency Level
	most recover spontaneously within 1–2 minutes.	

Cerebrovascular Disease is a Lifestyle Disease

When discussing the causes, cerebrovascular disease and the acute myocardial infarction we mentioned in the previous chapter are remarkably similar. People often discuss them together, referring to them as cardiovascular and cerebrovascular diseases. As mentioned earlier, coronary heart disease is related to atherosclerosis, and the same is true for cerebrovascular diseases.

The high-risk groups for cerebrovascular diseases are similar to those for coronary heart disease, primarily middle-aged and elderly individuals. These people generally have risk factors like hypertension, diabetes, dyslipidemia, smoking, obesity, staying up late, and high psychological stress. Additionally, people with habits of smoking and drinking are prone to cerebrovascular diseases, and high stress can also trigger its onset. Corporate executives, government officials, and white-collar workers are also high-risk groups.

For cerebrovascular diseases, aside from age, race, gender, and genetic factors, the most dangerous causative factors are hypertension, high blood sugar, and smoking.

The phrase "Smoking is harmful to health" seems universally understood, yet many people still don't take it seriously. Smoking directly damages endothelial cells of blood vessels, reducing the smoothness of the vessel walls, leading to cholesterol buildup and plaque formation. Most smokers have problems with atherosclerosis, which is the pathological basis for acute cerebrovascular diseases and coronary heart disease.

Emergency Scene

I have a friend named Ye Zhiping. Many people might not recognize his name, but if you mention the "most incredible principal" during the 2008 Wenchuan Earthquake, people will know. He was the principal of Sangzao Middle School, leading over 2,000 teachers and students to safety with no casualties, creating a miracle.

Before the Wenchuan Earthquake, he used all the funds allocated to the school to reinforce the school buildings. At that time, many teachers disagreed, but he persisted. When the earthquake struck, he was outside, not at the school, and rushed back. When he arrived, he saw that none of the school buildings had collapsed. All 2,000 students were gathered in the middle of the playground, surrounded by over 100 teachers, who were protecting them, all safe and sound. Overwhelmed with emotion, Principal Ye sat on the ground and burst into tears.

Ye Zhiping was a native of Sichuan, not very tall, and always had a cigarette in his mouth. He smoked two packs a day, had emphysema, spoke with a wheeze, and had a blood pressure over 200 but still refused to take medication. After the Wenchuan Earthquake, he became famous instantly. Even Premier Wen met with him to discuss future plans. The school received donations worth hundreds of millions of yuan, keeping him extremely busy. Many people also called him to donate more money or items. He said, "I don't need them anymore. I already have several vehicles. Thanks, but no more. I don't need money either. I have a few hundred million now, more than enough for a small middle school!" I was very familiar with him, so I joked, "Don't refuse them! Give it to me instead."

Of course, this was a joke. In fact, I was more concerned about his health than his career. Every time we met, I urged him to quit smoking and to visit the hospital, but he never listened. He was just like me—carefree and indifferent to everything. The last time we met was in October 2010, when we were invited to Xi'an to train dozens of principals on campus safety. His wheezing had worsened, and he even ate fatty meat during meals. I told him, "You really need to change your lifestyle. If you keep ignoring my advice, you'll either have a stroke or heart failure sooner or later!" Because we were so close, I didn't hold back my words. He just laughed it off and didn't take it to heart.

As expected, on June 27, 2011, he suffered a cerebral hemorrhage and couldn't be resuscitated. His passing was heartbreaking, as it resulted from his unhealthy lifestyle.

The best way to prevent cerebrovascular disease is to immediately change unhealthy lifestyle habits and undergo regular medical check-ups, thus preventing issues before they arise. As the saying goes, many illnesses are "eaten into existence." In the past, when people couldn't even afford enough to eat, there were few cases of cerebrovascular diseases. But now, it's not just the middle-aged and elderly who suffer from them; even young people are increasingly affected. Therefore, to stay away from and prevent cerebrovascular diseases, one must watch their diet and exercise regularly. By maintaining a healthy lifestyle, many dangerous diseases can be avoided or minimized.

Stay away from sudden cerebrovascular injury

Category	Details
Diet Management	- Eat more fresh vegetables and fruits daily: at least 400g of vegetables and 100-200g of fruits. - Eat fish 2-3 times a week, especially sea fish, and try to reduce animal meat intake. - Avoid too much oil or fat daily. - Reduce salt, alcohol, and coffee intake: no more than 6g of salt per day; men should not consume more than 50g of alcohol (1 bottle of beer) daily, women half of that amount. - Drink tea regularly. - Stick to the "three lows" principle in diet: low salt, low fat, low sugar.
Exercise	- Engage in light activities 20 minutes after meals, such as walking or Tai Chi. - If physically fit, choose aerobic activities such as running, cycling,

Category	Details
	swimming, etc., and keep up long-term consistency.
Other Precautions	- Avoid cold weather or when temperatures fluctuate between hot and cold. Avoid outdoor activities when it's too cold. - Keep your living environment at a suitable temperature and humidity, ensuring comfort. - Avoid overly hot or cold showers, especially for the elderly.

Eating more fresh vegetables and fruits is beneficial.

Vegetables and fruits are rich in vitamins, especially Vitamin C and beta-carotene, as well as minerals like calcium, phosphorus, potassium, and magnesium, plus dietary fiber. Regular consumption can reduce cholesterol, enhance vascular elasticity, promote myocardial enzyme metabolism, and protect cerebral vascular health, which is much better than relying on medication. It is recommended to eat no less than 400 grams of fresh vegetables and 100-200 grams of fruits daily. Opt for fresh, dark green vegetables and fruits such as strawberries, oranges, and kiwi.

Protein is also essential. It is recommended to eat fish 2-3 times a week, especially marine fish, which contain unsaturated fatty acids that help improve vascular elasticity and permeability, regulate blood pressure, reduce the incidence of cerebrovascular disease, and inhibit thrombosis. Other sources like milk and tofu are also good options. Try to avoid eating animal organs such as liver, kidneys, and fish roe.

Pay attention to portion control and avoid excessive fat intake. Eating too much food can convert into blood lipids, leading to elevated lipid levels. Over time, this can lead to high blood pressure and arteriosclerosis. Most people who suffer from cerebrovascular disease tend to be overweight and not physically active, making it even more crucial to avoid consuming too much fat, such as fatty meat, cream, and fried foods.

Reduce salt, alcohol, and coffee intake. Excessive salt intake can easily cause high blood pressure, which can then lead to cerebrovascular disease. Daily salt intake should be limited to about 6 grams (equivalent to the volume of a beer bottle cap). This is especially important for those who prefer salty foods. Alcohol can cause blood vessels to dilate, speeding up blood flow and increasing cerebral blood flow, which is why some people experience acute brain hemorrhage after drinking. Therefore, alcohol consumption should be limited: men should not exceed 50 grams of spirits or 1 bottle of beer daily, and women should have half of this amount. Pregnant women should avoid alcohol altogether. As for coffee, its stimulant properties can cause cerebral vasoconstriction, reducing cerebral blood flow over time, leading to ischemia, dizziness, and increased risk of disease.

Stick to a "three low" diet—low oil, low salt, and low sugar—to combat "three high conditions"— high blood lipids, high blood pressure, and high blood sugar.

Additionally, physical activity is very beneficial for preventing and improving cerebrovascular diseases. After resting for 20 minutes post-meal, take a walk or practice Tai Chi. Those in good physical condition can choose brisk walking, jogging, cycling, swimming, and other activities.

Weather changes significantly affect cerebrovascular disease onset. During hot summer days, many people may feel chest tightness and shortness of breath, while in extremely cold winters, blood vessels are prone to contraction. Extreme heat or cold can negatively impact cerebral blood vessels, potentially triggering acute cerebrovascular diseases. Therefore, if there are cerebrovascular patients or high-risk individuals in the family, it's important for family members to closely monitor their health during weather changes. During extremely cold or hot days or sudden temperature fluctuations, avoid letting patients engage in outdoor activities. The indoor environment should be kept at a comfortable and stable temperature and humidity level. Additionally, elderly patients should avoid saunas and instead take showers at home. This not only avoids the high temperature and humidity of saunas, which may be detrimental to the elderly but also helps prevent accidents such as falls or fainting.

Another important note: Patients with cerebrovascular diseases should avoid intense emotional stimulation, especially older patients.

Emergency Case

I've encountered some older patients who, during moments of intense excitement, experienced increased heart rate and blood pressure, triggering medical emergencies.

Once, I received an emergency call about an older gentleman who had collapsed, urging me to rush over. Upon arrival, he was lying in bed, dressed in thermal underwear, with a wet spot near his genital area.

At that time, I noticed he was semi-conscious— he could feel pain when pinched, furrowed his brows, and could still move his hands. I asked the elderly woman next to him, "What happened?"

She replied, "This is my husband. He asked me to manually stimulate him, then suddenly jerked and ended up like this. At first, I thought he was just feeling good, but when he didn't respond or wake up, I realized something was wrong and called 120 immediately."

This patient had a history of high blood pressure, and upon examination, he already exhibited partial limb paralysis and facial paralysis, with a blood pressure of 200/120 mmHg. Initially, it was suspected to be a cerebral hemorrhage. I immediately administered mannitol to reduce intracranial pressure and lower his elevated blood pressure before rushing him to the hospital. A CT scan confirmed a brain hemorrhage.

High blood pressure, in itself, is not too concerning, but it can damage vital organs. When subjected to strong stimuli, the sudden spike in blood pressure can cause dizziness, headaches, or in severe cases, cerebral hemorrhage.

From this example, it is clear that elderly individuals should exercise caution during sexual activity. Of course, the sexual activity itself is only a trigger; the main cause remains high blood pressure.

Before the arrival of emergency services (120), the most important task is to prevent asphyxiation.

For stroke (cerebral infarction) patients, thrombolysis within 3 hours is the most effective, with earlier treatment leading to better outcomes. After a blood clot forms, the brain tissue surrounding the infarcted area only temporarily loses function. If blood vessels can be reopened and blood supply restored quickly, this part of the brain tissue may be saved from necrosis. Delaying even a minute reduces the speed and degree of recovery for stroke patients: time is critical in treating cerebrovascular disease.

To prevent the tongue from falling back in a supine position, and to avoid choking on vomit or secretions, the rescuer should place the patient in a "stable side-lying position". If there is vomit, secretions, dentures, or other foreign objects in the patient's mouth, they should be cleared immediately.

If the patient is conscious, provide reassurance, keep the environment quiet to reduce their anxiety, and avoid exposing them to strong light. Ensure good air circulation, and if oxygen is available, administer it to the patient. Do not give the patient any medication until a doctor has made a clear diagnosis.

You can also perform some simple checks, such as calling the patient's name to see if they can respond, or checking their blood pressure with a blood pressure monitor and keeping a record.

Avoid moving the patient unnecessarily to prevent worsening their condition. If moving the patient is essential, the correct method is for one person to support the head and shoulders, another to support the back and hips, and a third to lift the waist and legs. Working together, gently lift the patient onto a hard wooden board or stretcher, ensuring the movement is horizontal. Do not carry, drag, or lift the patient over your shoulder or back.

Different cerebrovascular symptoms require

specific handling methods, so it's important to consider the patient's unique situation.

How to deal with patients in coma, shock, and syncope?

Condition	Guidelines
Coma	1. Keep the patient calm, ensure absolute bed rest, stabilize the head, and avoid unnecessary movements. 2. Ensure the patient's airway is clear, do not give water, medication, or food; position in a "stable side-lying position". 3. Call emergency services (120) immediately. 4. Transfer quickly to a hospital with CT scanning facilities.
Convulsions	1. Immediately place the patient flat, stabilize the head, and maintain calmness. 2. Ensure the patient's airway is unobstructed to prevent suffocation. 3. Regardless of the weather,

Condition	Guidelines
	keep the patient warm.
	4. Call emergency services (120) immediately, and if oxygen is available, provide it to the patient.
Syncope (Fainting)	Place the patient flat. Do not shake or lift them up; they will typically regain consciousness after 1-2 minutes.

Unconscious Patient: Ensuring an Open Airway is Crucial

First, keep the patient calm and ensure they remain strictly in bed. Avoid using high pillows to prevent pressure on the blood vessels. Additionally, avoid unnecessary movement, especially any jarring of the head.

Second, the most important thing is to ensure the patient's airway remains open. For unconscious patients, place them in the "stable side-lying position."

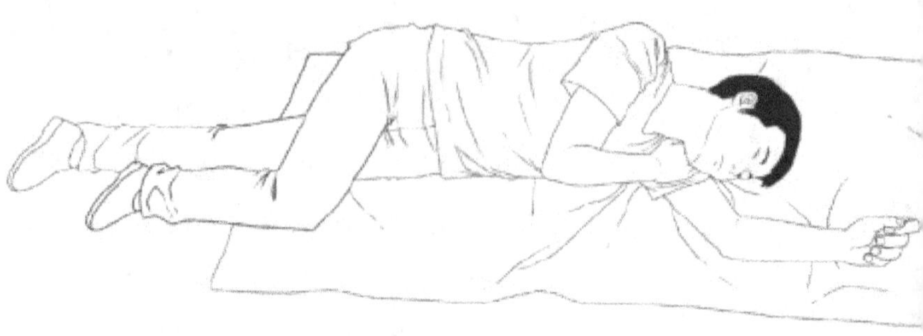

Also, clear the patient's mouth of vomit, secretions, dentures, or other foreign objects. Be sure not to give the patient water or medication, even if they seem conscious. Why? Because in patients with acute cerebrovascular disease, their swallowing function may be impaired. Not only unconscious patients, but even conscious ones with hemiplegia may accidentally swallow the medication into the airway, which can be dangerous. There was once an elderly patient who had an acute cerebrovascular attack, and in the family's panic, they noticed the patient's blood pressure rising and immediately gave them antihypertensive medication and water. Tragically, the patient choked to death.

Third, immediately call emergency services at 120.

Fourth, get to a hospital with a CT scanner

quickly to determine whether the patient is experiencing a hemorrhage or ischemia, which part of the brain is affected, the amount of bleeding, and the extent of brain tissue necrosis. Once this is determined, the doctors can provide targeted treatment accordingly.

Shock Patient: Keep the Patient Warm

First, lay the patient flat and, if there's a pillow, remove it immediately. Keep the patient calm; the goal is to ensure sufficient blood flow to the brain and buy valuable time until medical personnel arrive.

Second, make sure the patient's airway is open to prevent asphyxiation from vomiting or other causes.

Third, a commonly overlooked point: keeping the patient warm. Even during the hottest summer days, people in shock often feel cold because their microcirculation is impaired.

Fourth, if oxygen is available, let the patient inhale it immediately, and of course, call emergency services at 120.

Fainting Patient: Simply Lay Them Flat

If a patient faints, the treatment is much simpler—just lay the patient flat. Once flat, blood flow to the brain will quickly restore, and the patient will soon regain consciousness. Some suggest pinching the philtrum when someone faints, but this doesn't actually help. Fainting typically resolves on its own, and the patient will wake up within a minute or two.

In the past, in old Beijing, people often bathed at public bathhouses, where groups of men soaked in pools, and fainting incidents were common after soaking for too long.

Once, at the Hufangqiao Bathhouse, someone called emergency services saying a 70-year-old man had fainted in the pool. We happened to be nearby, so we turned around and headed there. When we arrived, the elderly man had already been lifted onto a bench and was lying down, surrounded by a crowd. Before we could even examine him, someone from the bathhouse came over with a glass of cold water, took a big gulp, and sprayed it all over the elderly man's face. He immediately woke up, dazed, but got up feeling fine. Upon further examination, we found nothing wrong with him; it was just a simple fainting episode. This was caused by the elderly man's brain receiving insufficient blood supply. The person at the bathhouse had used a traditional folk remedy—spraying cold water to wake him up. In fact, if they had just left him alone, laying him flat and ensuring sufficient blood supply to the brain, he would have woken up on his own.

After regaining consciousness, most fainting patients feel fine, except for some weakness, dizziness, or heart palpitations. At this point, check their pulse and blood pressure. If the patient is otherwise fine, with normal limb movements and clear speech, there's generally nothing to worry about. However, if the heart rate speeds up or slows down, reaching above 120 or below 60 beats per minute, this could be cardiogenic syncope, and you must immediately call emergency services and get professional medical treatment.

Symptoms of a cerebrovascular attack vary in severity, and not everyone will lose consciousness. However, you should never be complacent. If you feel unwell, seek medical attention as soon as possible, because being conscious doesn't necessarily mean there's no brain tissue damage. Many stroke patients remain conscious throughout the attack but later find their mouth drooping, limbs unresponsive, or speech slurred. While it may not be life-threatening, it can leave long-term effects, so it's important to stay vigilant.

How Should First Aid Be Administered? Should You Help an Elderly Person Who Has Fallen?

Speaking of laying down a fainted patient flat, it reminds me of a hot topic in recent years—whether to help an elderly person who has fallen. Nowadays, when an elderly person falls, a crowd of onlookers often gathers, but few people offer assistance. Even when someone tries to help, they are often "kindly" discouraged by others, leading to several tragedies.

This issue—whether to help a fallen elderly person—has become not only a medical question but also a societal issue. After the Ministry of Health released the *Elderly Fall Intervention Technical Guidelines*, several media outlets interviewed me to ask for my opinion, and many netizens have also inquired about what to do in such situations. My answer is: Regardless of the circumstances, if you see an elderly person fall, do not hastily try to help them up; you should first ask questions and check their condition.

Upon hearing this, some might say I lack compassion. But it's not about lacking compassion—it's about assessing the situation carefully. In many cases, providing first aid on the spot is more important than immediately helping someone to their feet. When you see an elderly person fall, regardless of the cause—whether they tripped, felt dizzy, or were hit by a vehicle—the first step is to check their consciousness by asking, "Are you okay?" If there's no response, the person is unconscious. Next, check their breathing. If they aren't breathing, immediately begin cardiopulmonary resuscitation (CPR). If they are breathing, place them in the "stable side-lying position" to maintain a clear airway, and then call emergency services.

How to help an elderly person who has fallen down?

At the Scene of First Aid

Speaking of this, I recall a rather awkward incident involving sudden death that I once encountered.

Once, we arrived at a patient's home and found two elderly people in bed, one on top of the other, covered by a blanket. When we lifted the blanket, both of them were completely naked, with the old man lying on top of the old woman. We immediately understood: the elderly couple had just been having intercourse.

I quickly checked the old man and found that he had no heartbeat or breathing, and his lips were cyanotic. The old woman, on the other hand, was fine; she lay underneath, wide-eyed and afraid to move.

Upon further inquiry, we learned that the old man had taken Viagra that evening, became overly excited, and had a seizure at the moment of ejaculation, after which he collapsed on top of the old woman. At first, the old woman thought it was just a normal sexual climax, but after a while, she sensed something was wrong as he wasn't responding to her calls or any shaking. Realizing the urgency, she called for help. Their children soon arrived but didn't dare move him. They just covered the couple with a blanket and immediately called emergency services, not knowing what else to do, standing around in shock until we arrived.

I then asked the children, "This man is already gone, why didn't you move him off?" After a long pause, they hesitantly replied, "Isn't it dangerous to move someone with heart disease?"

Hearing this, I was quite frustrated. I thought to myself: If someone there had understood the situation even a little, had moved him off quickly and started CPR while calling emergency services, there might have been a chance to save him.

Therefore, the question of whether to assist someone who has fallen should be based on the specific situation. Don't recklessly assist, but also don't stand by and miss the opportunity for rescue.

The elderly man in this example died from what is known as "sudden death during intercourse," which refers to sudden, accidental death triggered by sexual activity. Death is something no one wishes to experience, yet it is something we all must face and accept. It's especially tragic when death occurs unexpectedly while enjoying life. Sudden death during intercourse is one of the most ironic forms of sudden death. So, it's important to be cautious during sexual activity—don't overexert yourself, control your excitement, and know your limits. This is especially true for the elderly, those with illnesses, those who are overly tired, drunk, or who have taken aphrodisiacs. People with high blood pressure or coronary heart disease need to be particularly careful.

Another somewhat special situation involves patients with cerebrovascular disease who collapse due to an epileptic seizure.

We occasionally encounter patients having a major seizure. Cerebrovascular disease is an important cause of secondary epilepsy. Epilepsy, often called "yangjiao feng" or "yangxian feng" in Chinese, affects 8 to 9 million people in China. Families with a history of epilepsy generally have experience and know that the patient's life is not in danger, waiting until the convulsions stop before taking them to the hospital. However, during a major seizure, the patient suddenly collapses, foaming at the mouth and convulsing, which can be quite terrifying for those witnessing it for the first time. What should you do in such a situation?

Should you help? Can you help? To be honest, during a seizure, you don't really need to help them up, and it's actually quite difficult to do so.

When we emergency doctors encounter a seizure patient, what do we generally do? I usually loosen the patient's collar and administer diazepam. Once the seizure subsides and the condition stabilizes, we transport the patient to the hospital.

For most people, family members likely don't have diazepam on hand, nor would they carry it with them. In such cases, what you can do is loosen the patient's collar to ensure their airway is clear. Avoid forcibly restraining the patient; let them convulse freely, and call emergency services immediately. After the seizure stops, place the patient in a stable side-lying position and wait for the ambulance to arrive.

Some readers may have heard or read elsewhere that when someone is having a seizure, you should put something between their teeth to prevent them from biting their tongue. In practice, however, this is very difficult to do. During a seizure, the patient's jaws are clenched, making it nearly impossible to insert anything. Forcing something into their mouth could easily damage their teeth.

As family members, when you first encounter a seizure, you might lack experience, but after several occurrences, you'll know to be more cautious. If you notice the patient's condition suddenly worsening, you should immediately support them and gently lay them on the ground to prevent injury from the fall.

The seizure itself may not cause significant harm to the patient, but the fall during the seizure could result in various external injuries.

Chapter 4: Trauma - First Aid Has Guidelines to Follow

First Aid Awareness Can Save Lives – Don't Fear "Overreacting"

At the Scene of First Aid

1.

Many years ago, the Beijing Emergency Center received a call about an injured foreigner at the International Machine Tool Exhibition, and we were asked to rush over. When we arrived, we saw a tall foreign man lying on the ground. His expression showed no sign of pain, and his eyes were on us—he was fully conscious but completely immobile. Those around him informed me that he was a representative from a Danish company. While operating a machine tool during a demonstration, the tool suddenly flew out. Fortunately, his reflexes were quick, and he dodged the tool in time, avoiding being hit. However, he lost his balance and fell to the ground, where he remained.

I asked the translator, "Why hasn't he gotten up

after all this time?"

The translator conveyed my question, and the man responded with something that shocked me: "I'll only get up if the doctor tells me to." I had never heard a Chinese person say anything like that before. His words showed how much trust foreigners place in doctors. This approach is also scientific—if someone is truly injured, moving without understanding the nature of the injury could worsen it.

I immediately examined him from head to toe and found no issues. I asked, "How are you feeling now?"

He said, "I don't feel bad."

I then asked, "Can you stand up by yourself?"

He replied, "Are you a doctor?"

When the translator informed him that I was a doctor from the Beijing Emergency Center, he finally stood up.

This incident had a big impact on me. Foreigners receive first aid education from a young age and have this kind of awareness, but most Chinese people lack it. If we fall, most of us immediately assume we're fine if nothing seems broken and get up right away. We would never lie on the ground in the same position for so long. To the Chinese onlookers, the foreigner's behavior seemed like an overreaction, even a bit "foolish." But was he really overreacting? In fact, the real "foolishness" lies with us. Let me share another story to explain.

2.

One day, a bus was driving down the road when suddenly, a bicycle swerved into the lane from the bike path. Right at that critical moment, there was a large bus coming from the opposite direction, and the driver had no choice but to slam on the brakes. Fortunately, the bus stopped just half a meter behind the bike, but the sudden and forceful braking caused some passengers standing at the back to lurch forward. A man in his 50s fell to the floor but quickly got up. The driver turned and asked, "Is anyone hurt?" Everyone, including the man who fell, said no.

The driver, in a hurry, cursed the cyclist and continued driving.

A few minutes later, the man who had fallen began to experience abdominal pain and bloating, and suddenly collapsed on the floor, his face pale and covered in cold sweat. The driver, panicking, pulled over to the side of the road and immediately called emergency services at 120.

When we arrived, we boarded the bus and saw the patient curled up on the floor, his face pale—showing signs of acute anemia and typical symptoms of hemorrhagic shock. The driver, still nervous, quickly explained the situation. While listening, I examined the patient's abdomen. When I pressed on his abdomen, the pain worsened, and when I released the pressure, the pain intensified again. His abdomen felt hard, and his muscles were very tense ("rebound tenderness, abdominal guarding" are three main signs of peritoneal irritation). When I checked his blood pressure, it was 60/40 mmHg.

Considering his injury history and the signs of peritoneal irritation and shock, it was clear that his abdominal organs were bleeding. I immediately established two intravenous lines to rapidly replenish blood volume, and we rushed him to Beijing Jishuitan Hospital for further diagnosis and treatment.

Two days later, when I was back at the hospital delivering another patient, I spoke to the surgeon who had treated the shock patient. He told me, "Dr. Jia, the patient you brought in with abdominal bleeding underwent exploratory surgery soon after arrival. The result was a ruptured mesenteric artery with significant bleeding. We performed a ligation, blood transfusion, and anti-shock measures. Thankfully, he arrived early and we saved him."

How did the mesenteric artery rupture? It was due to the sudden force from braking, which caused the entire body to lurch forward abruptly, and the mesenteric artery was violently pulled and torn. This is a classic example of a concealed injury with delayed symptoms, often overlooked.

After hearing this story, many people probably won't mock that Danish man for "overreacting." These situations, which may seem like overreactions or unnecessary fuss to us, actually make a lot of sense. As the saying goes, "It's better to believe there's a problem than to assume there isn't"—being cautious in critical moments could save a life.

The Danish man is a great example of how their approach to first aid is far superior to ours in many respects. It's something we should definitely learn from.

Don't Move After an Injury – No External Wounds Doesn't Mean No Internal Damage

In martial arts novels, there are often scenes like this: a powerful martial artist strikes with an intense blow, and although the person hit shows no signs of injury on the surface, they suddenly cough up blood and collapse, dead from internal organs being shattered by the force of the blow.

Of course, in real life, we won't encounter such "martial arts masters." But from a medical perspective, is there anything remotely similar? Yes.

At the Scene of First Aid

I know a high school teacher who once went on a trip organized by the school. While they were descending a mountain, the bus's brakes failed, and the vehicle tumbled down the mountain. Everyone on board was thrown out of the windows with force. There were over 60 people on the bus, and more than a dozen died on the spot. It was a major accident.

One of the teachers was thrown out of the bus but managed to get up, stretch his limbs, and felt that he wasn't seriously hurt since there were no external injuries. He didn't think much of it. Being kind-hearted, he immediately started helping others escape danger. He continued helping for over half an hour. When the emergency vehicle arrived, he sighed in relief and sat down, thinking he could finally rest. But as soon as he sat down, his face turned as pale as paper, and after collapsing, he never got back up. He died right there. Later, when he was taken to the hospital for an examination, it was found that he had died from internal organ injuries leading to chronic internal bleeding. If he hadn't moved around so much, he might have lessened the severity of his injuries, and there might have been a chance to save him at the hospital.

Human beings are made of flesh and blood, and when subjected to extreme external force, it's very possible for internal organs to be "shattered." Cases of internal injuries due to violent external trauma often occur in traffic accidents. When traffic accidents happen, the victims frequently suffer severe and complex injuries due to the immense force involved, often leading to multiple organ and body part damage. The most dangerous part is that these "internal injuries" tend to be concealed and not immediately apparent, which can delay medical treatment or lead to the victim unknowingly moving around, exacerbating internal bleeding—leaving them with deep regret afterward.

So, how can you tell if a victim is suffering from external bleeding, internal bleeding, or subcutaneous bleeding? It's actually quite simple:

Which is more dangerous, internal or external bleeding? Most people believe external bleeding is more dangerous, as the victims who die on the spot are usually those suffering from severe external bleeding. On the other hand, patients with internal bleeding, such as intracranial hemorrhage or ruptured liver or spleen, often make it to the hospital in time.

However, the truth is that internal bleeding is more dangerous and harder to treat than external bleeding. External bleeding, such as from a knife wound, cut, or animal bite, is easier to manage. Even if someone isn't a doctor, they can often handle such injuries themselves after some basic training. Internal bleeding, on the other hand, is much more difficult to treat and is nearly impossible to address outside of a hospital. For example, if someone has a ruptured liver, even the best hepatobiliary surgeon in China couldn't perform surgery on the street. Generally speaking, if you suspect that someone has internal bleeding, don't move them, and don't let them move. This will prevent the bleeding from worsening. Additionally, don't give them water, as it could lead to vomiting during surgery, which could cause choking. Just keep them still and wait quietly for the ambulance to arrive.

Correctly distinguish between external bleeding,

internal bleeding and subcutaneous bleeding

Type of Bleeding	Description
External Bleeding	Typically caused by sharp objects, such as being cut by a knife. Blood flows out through the skin or mucous membranes, resulting in visible external bleeding.
Internal Bleeding	Caused by external force acting on the body, resulting in damage to deep tissues or organs. Blood does not flow out through the skin or mucous membranes (e.g., liver rupture). There is no visible blood flow on the surface of the skin.
Subcutaneous Bleeding	The injured area becomes bruised and swollen. Similar to internal bleeding, subcutaneous bleeding does not show any visible blood flow on the surface of the skin.

Arterial Bleeding: Apply Firm Pressure

Asphyxiation, severe bleeding, and serious internal organ damage are the top three causes of early death. The causes of asphyxiation vary, and the methods and difficulty of treatment differ. When it comes to severe internal organ damage, there's not much that can be done at the scene—it's essential to get to the hospital as quickly as possible for emergency treatment. However, for severe bleeding, timely and effective control of bleeding is often the key to saving a life, and learning how to stop bleeding is something anyone can master quickly with practical use in emergency situations.

A person's blood volume typically makes up 7% to 8% of their body weight, usually calculated as 8%. For example, a person weighing 50 kilograms has about 4,000 milliliters of blood. When 20% of the total blood volume is lost, shock occurs. When 40% of the total blood volume is lost, life is in danger. Therefore, stopping bleeding promptly and effectively at the scene is the most crucial step in saving a life.

At the Scene of First Aid

One evening in the mid-1980s, as darkness fell, a "yellow wind" blew through the city—it was what we now call a sandstorm. The wind was strong, carrying dust that made it hard to open your eyes. After work, I stopped by a foreign-language bookstore near Bamiancao to browse, parking my bike at the entrance. After finishing, as I was preparing to leave, I suddenly saw a window guard panel fall straight from above and strike a woman in her 30s on the head as she passed by. She collapsed immediately, and blood sprayed over a meter into the air—it all happened in an instant.

I immediately abandoned my bike by the roadside and ran across the street. By this time, the injured woman was unconscious, being held by a passerby, but the blood was still gushing. I quickly pulled out a clean handkerchief from my pocket, folded it a few times, and applied firm pressure to the gushing wound with one hand. With my other hand, I pressed my thumb on her superficial temporal artery. The fountain-like bleeding stopped immediately.

At this point, several other bystanders stepped in to help. We flagged down a small "bengbeng" (a type of motorized tricycle), and with everyone's effort, we lifted the injured woman onto the vehicle and all rode along with her.

On the way to Peking Union Medical College Hospital, I felt the wound through the handkerchief and found that the skull on the right side of her head was depressed—indicating a skull fracture.

After dropping off the injured woman, I returned to the bookstore to retrieve my bike, where I found a man in his 60s sitting nearby. He said, "Young man, is this your bike? You forgot to lock it in your rush to help. I've been watching it for you." I was deeply moved. Despite the cold weather and the fierce wind, this elderly man with gray hair had been guarding my bike.

Nowadays, when we're debating whether or not to help an elderly person who has fallen, well… sigh.

The next day, while delivering a patient to Peking Union Medical College Hospital, I inquired about the condition of the injured woman. The nurse on duty said, "The woman from yesterday had a depressed skull fracture and significant bleeding. Thankfully, a few kind-hearted people got her to the hospital in time, and I heard that a doctor from an emergency station was passing by after work and promptly applied measures to stop the bleeding. She's been saved."

If no one had applied pressure to stop the bleeding at the scene, the woman would likely have gone into shock very quickly, putting her life at risk. Arterial bleeding is characterized by bright red blood spurting from the proximal wound in a pulsating manner, making it extremely dangerous. In contrast, venous bleeding is darker red, with blood continuously oozing from the distal wound, making it relatively less dangerous than arterial bleeding. However, large venous ruptures can still be very dangerous.

Simply put, if you see blood spurting out, it's a clear sign of arterial rupture and bleeding. There's also capillary bleeding, which is when the surface of the skin is scratched, and blood oozes out slowly. This type of bleeding is common in everyday life with small scrapes, and there's no danger—people can handle it themselves, so we won't go into detail here.

Now, some might wonder, "With such heavy bleeding like that woman had, does pressing down on the artery really work?" For head injuries, bleeding from ruptured arteries above the eyebrows, on the forehead, or on the sides of the head can be controlled by pressing on the superficial temporal artery. For bleeding from the occipital artery, pressure on the occipital artery is needed to stop the bleeding.

But what about heavy bleeding from other parts of the body—where should you apply pressure?

If I were giving a demonstration in person, everyone would clearly understand the locations of the pressure points. However, for the average person, in an emergency, it's not easy to quickly and accurately locate these points. The general principle of pressure-based bleeding control is as follows: For heavy arterial bleeding in the lower limbs, use your fist to press firmly at the root of the thigh, which is the proximal location of the femoral artery. If the bleeding is from the lower leg, you can press either the femoral artery or the popliteal artery. The popliteal artery is located at the junction of the lower leg and thigh, behind the knee. Similarly, for upper limb injuries, press at the root of the arm or use your thumb to press on the subclavian artery. Not many people know about the subclavian artery, but if the arm or hand is cut, pressing this artery can help stop the bleeding. For limb bleeding, it's usually easy to follow the bleeding site to find the blood vessel and apply pressure at the proximal end to stop the bleeding.

While pressure-based bleeding control for major arterial bleeding is immediately effective, it does have a drawback—it cannot be maintained for long periods. After applying pressure for a while, your hands will tire, and the pressure will weaken, reducing the effectiveness of the bleeding control. Therefore, after pressing on the bleeding point, if the situation becomes less critical, quickly find something to use for bandaging.

How to Stop Arterial Bleeding?

1. Direct Pressure on the Bleeding Site
This is the most commonly used, easiest to master, fastest, and most effective immediate method of bleeding control in emergency first aid. It can be applied to arterial, venous, and capillary bleeding.

1. Cover the wound with a dressing, handkerchief, or similar material.

2. Then, press firmly on the wound using your fingers or palm. After a few minutes, the bleeding should typically stop.

3. Once the bleeding stops, apply a pressure bandage.

2. Pressure Point Bleeding Control

Although the pressure point method is somewhat harder for the average person to master, it can still be very effective in practice. For instance, if an artery in the upper limb is severed and blood is spurting out, you can use your thumb to press on the proximal end of the bleeding vessel (the proximal end is closer to the heart, while the distal end is farther from the heart). This compresses the blood vessel, stopping blood flow and achieving hemostasis.

Several commonly used hemostatic points on the body

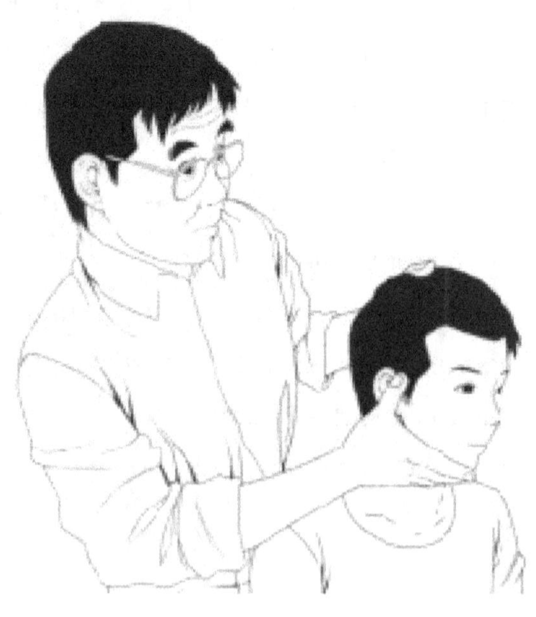

Hemostatic Point: Superficial Temporal Artery

Scope of Application: Arterial rupture and bleeding in the forehead, temporal region, or the top of the head.

Location: In the depression located above and in front of the tragus on both sides, where a pulse can be felt.

Hemostatic Point: Occipital Artery

Scope of Application: Arterial rupture and bleeding in the occipital region.

Location: In the depression between the sternocleidomastoid muscle and the trapezius muscle (below and behind the mastoid process).

Hemostatic Point: Carotid Artery

Scope of Application: Severe bleeding from a carotid artery rupture when other compression sites are ineffective.

Location: At the pulsating point on the inner edge of the sternocleidomastoid muscle.

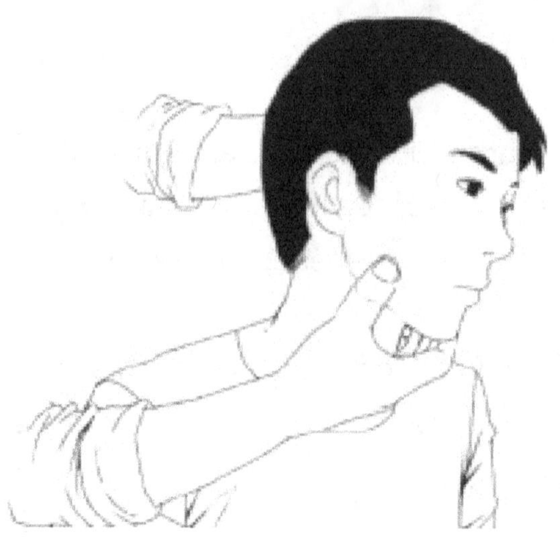

Hemostatic Point: Facial Artery

Scope of Application: Arterial rupture and bleeding in the maxillofacial region.

Location: 1.5 cm above and in front of the mandibular angle.

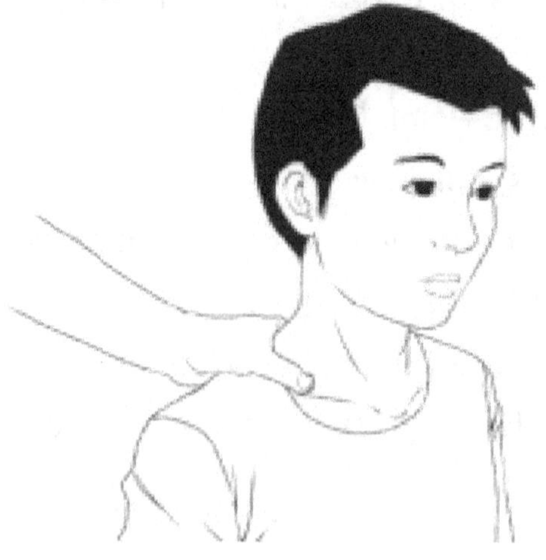

Hemostatic Point: Subclavian Artery

Scope of Application: Arterial rupture and bleeding in the shoulder, axilla, and upper limbs.
Location: At the pulsating point in the middle of the supraclavicular fossa.

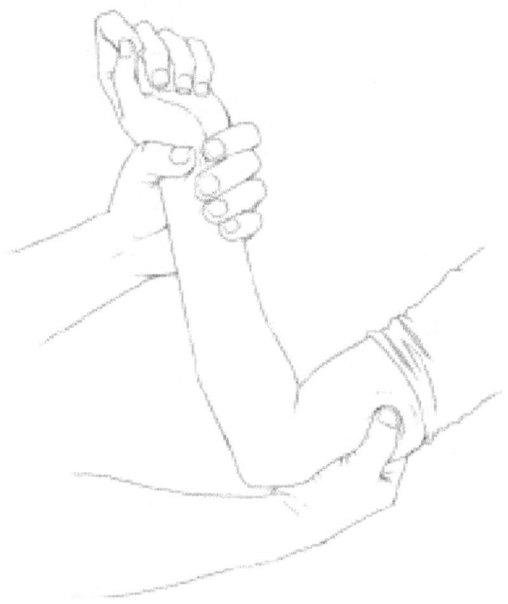

Hemostatic Point: Femoral Artery
Scope of Application: Severe arterial bleeding in the lower limbs.
Location: At the pulsating point just below the midpoint of the inguinal ligament.

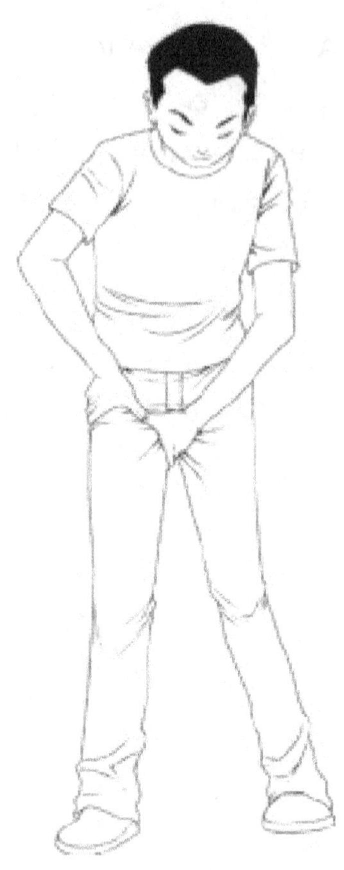

Hemostatic Point: Brachial Artery

Scope of Application: Arterial rupture and bleeding in the hand, forearm, and upper arm.

Location: At the pulsating point on the inner edge of the biceps brachii muscle of the upper arm.

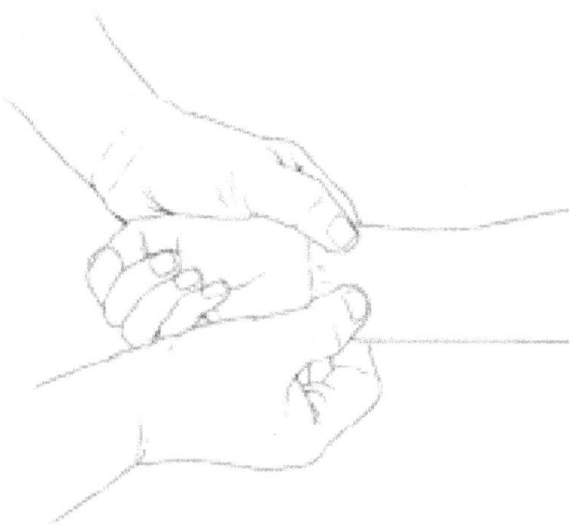

Hemostatic Point: Ulnar and Radial Arteries

Scope of Application: Arterial rupture and bleeding in the hand.

Location: At the pulsating points on both sides above the wrist crease.

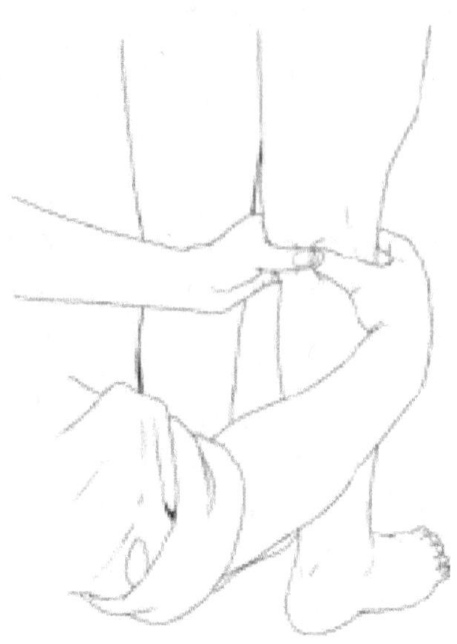

Hemostatic Point: Popliteal Artery

Scope of Application: Arterial rupture and bleeding in the lower leg and foot.

Location: At the pulsating point in the middle of the popliteal crease.

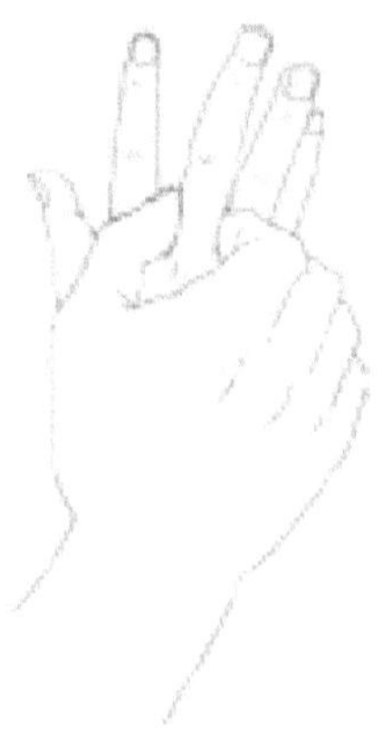

Hemostatic Point: Digital Arteries

Scope of Application: Arterial rupture and bleeding in the fingers.

Location: On both sides of the base of the finger.

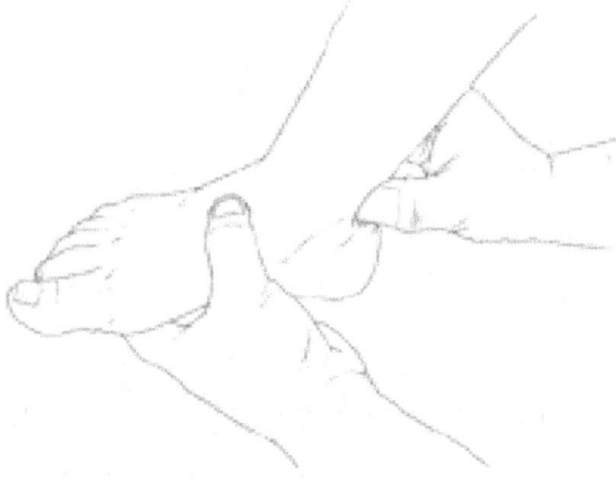

Hemostatic Point: Posterior Tibial Artery

Scope of Application: Arterial rupture and bleeding in the foot.

Location: Behind the medial malleolus (inner ankle).

Tourniquet: Life-saving when used correctly, harmful when misused

At the Scene of First Aid

One day in the 1970s, the Beijing cycling team was training on the highway. The team's formation was not in a straight line but staggered, following fluid mechanics or aerodynamic principles to reduce resistance and increase speed. Later, one of the cyclists in the rear moved into the fast lane, even riding against traffic.

At that moment, a car approached from the opposite direction, hitting the last cyclist. He was thrown off his bike, resulting in a complete open fracture of his right femur and complete rupture of the femoral artery, with blood spurting three to four meters away. It is important to know that a complete rupture of the femoral or carotid artery can lead to death from blood loss within 2 to 5 minutes. This young man was in critical condition!

The entire team stopped. Although team members were accustomed to minor injuries during training, no one had ever encountered such a severe situation before. They were all stunned, unsure of what to do. At this moment of extreme danger, the injured athlete suddenly sat up, overlapping his thumbs and pressing down hard on the femoral artery pressure point at the root of his thigh. Instantly, the spurting blood stopped.

Everyone was still in shock, but the young man loudly shouted to his teammates, "What are you waiting for? Get an inner tube!" His teammates immediately pulled out a bicycle inner tube, which made an excellent rubber tourniquet! They quickly tied the inner tube around the proximal end of the injury, effectively controlling the bleeding. The team breathed a sigh of relief, knowing that although he was seriously injured, he was no longer in immediate danger. They promptly called for an ambulance.

The athlete was later taken to the hospital for

surgery, and three months later, he was back in training, fully recovered.

This is a classic and astonishingly successful case of self-rescue and mutual aid!

This incident happened 35 years ago. At the time, I was working at the Beijing Institute of Sports Science. I heard this story firsthand from Mr. Wang Xingzhai, the team leader, while accompanying the Beijing football team for training at the Kunming Haigeng National Training Base. In the 1970s, Mr. Wang was the leader of the Beijing cycling team, and he personally witnessed this event. He was full of admiration for the young man involved.

Self-rescue and mutual aid require not only first-aid skills but also a mindset of awareness, wisdom, courage, agility, confidence, calmness, and decisiveness.

At that time, the athlete was in an extremely dangerous situation. If he had lacked first-aid knowledge and if no one around him knew how to help, he surely would have died. Here, I want to emphasize the importance of using a tourniquet correctly.

The Proper Use of a Tourniquet

Typically, the most ideal method of stopping bleeding is the use of a rubber tourniquet. A rubber tourniquet is a hollow rubber tube, 80 to 100 cm long. The rubber tube from a medical stethoscope is best suited for stopping bleeding in the upper limbs, while for the lower limbs, it should be doubled up to be effective.

Of course, we can't carry a rubber tourniquet with us all the time. So, what should we do in emergencies? If no rubber tourniquet is available, the twist-tourniquet method can be used. Materials such as triangular bandages, bed sheets, duvet covers, curtains, or tablecloths can be used, but non-elastic items like wire, electrical cords, or ropes should not be used as tourniquets.

How to Properly Use a Tourniquet:

1. Material Selection
If a professional tourniquet is not available, you can use elastic materials like triangular bandages, bed sheets, duvet covers, curtains, or tablecloths. Non-elastic items like wire, electrical cords, or ropes should not be used as tourniquets.

2. Tying Requirements
First, wrap the skin with a triangular bandage, towel, or clothing to create a smooth padding, and then tie the tourniquet around it.

3. Location Requirements
For the upper limbs, tie the tourniquet at the upper third of the arm. For the lower limbs, tie it around the middle of the thigh.

4. Tightness Requirements

Tighten the tourniquet until the bleeding stops or the distal arterial pulse disappears (the goal is to stop the bleeding with the minimum force necessary).

5. Time Requirements

Do not leave the tourniquet tied for more than 2 to 3 hours. Loosen it every 40 to 50 minutes. If there is bleeding after loosening, apply finger pressure for 5 to 10 minutes and then re-tie the tourniquet.

6. Marking

After tying the tourniquet, mark the time of application clearly at a visible spot and transport the injured person to the hospital as quickly as possible.

At the Scene of Another First Aid Incident

Once, at a construction site, a worker's hand

was cut deeply, severing an artery and causing significant bleeding. His coworkers used No. 8 lead wire (used for tying rebar) as a tourniquet and twisted it tightly with pliers. Then, they called our emergency center. By the time I arrived, the bleeding had stopped, but the worker's entire hand had turned black and purple. I quickly re-applied a rubber tourniquet and removed the lead wire with pliers. Fortunately, the time was short, and after hospital treatment, his hand recovered well. Had the wire been left on for too long, the worker's hand might have needed to be amputated.

In summary, using a tourniquet scientifically is crucial. When used correctly, it can save lives. However, incorrect use can lead to ischemia, muscle contraction, necrosis, nerve damage, or even kidney failure. When using a tourniquet, follow these important guidelines:

1. Do not tie the tourniquet directly on the skin. First, wrap a triangular bandage, towel, or clothing around the skin to prevent local injury.

2. Tie the tourniquet at the correct location. For the upper limbs, tie it at the upper third of the arm to avoid injuring the radial nerve. For the lower limbs, tie it at the middle of the thigh. Avoid tying it between bones, as there are interosseous arteries that make bleeding control less effective.

3. The tourniquet should be tight enough to stop the bleeding but not overly tight. If it is too tight, it may cause damage to nerves, blood vessels, and muscles; if it is too loose, it may only compress veins, leading to arterial bleeding without venous return, which can exacerbate shock or even be life-threatening.

4. Do not leave the tourniquet on for more than 3 hours. Loosen it every 40 to 50 minutes to temporarily restore blood flow to the distal limb. If bleeding resumes after loosening, use finger pressure to stop the bleeding for 5 to 10 minutes, then reapply the tourniquet slightly below the original spot.

5. After applying the tourniquet, clearly mark the time and promptly transport the injured person to a hospital for treatment.

Small Vessel Bleeding: Press Where It Bleeds

At the Scene of First Aid

I remember one summer, during an unbearably hot day, at Xiaochang Wutiao outside Xuanwumen, a young man from Shaanxi who delivered bottled water got into a conflict with someone. He pulled out a fruit knife and tried to stab them. However, the other side had three people, and the knife was quickly taken away and used to stab him instead.

There were a lot of bystanders, but no one knew what to do. So, everyone stood aside, talking and arguing among themselves, but no one helped the young man. Fortunately, someone eventually called for an ambulance. By the time I arrived, the attacker had long fled, and the injured man had already been taken to Guangnei Hospital by his fellow villagers. All that was left at the scene was a large pool of blood, thick and already coagulated.

When I reached Guangnei Hospital, the young man was lying in bed, wearing sports shorts with several layers of bandages wrapped around his right upper arm. He had already stopped breathing, and his heart had stopped beating. Upon unwrapping the bandages, I saw that the bleeding had stopped. There was only one wound on the inner side of his right upper arm, less than a centimeter in size. I examined his entire body and found no other injuries.

Could such a small wound have caused his death? Or was there another reason I hadn't discovered? It wasn't clear, but in any case, unnatural deaths are the responsibility of the police.

A few days later, detectives from the Xicheng District Public Security Bureau came to the emergency center to investigate the case. I shared everything I had seen and heard with them. The police also showed me a report from the Beijing Public Security Bureau's Forensic Center, which included a photo. In the photo was the young man's right arm, with a ruler placed beside it. The report stated, "Complete rupture of the brachial artery, 7 mm wound, death by hemorrhagic shock."

I felt it was such a tragedy—a 7 mm wound had taken the life of a strong young man.

In fact, at that time, if someone had immediately applied direct pressure to the young man's wound or compressed the artery proximal to the wound, the bleeding could have been stopped, and his life saved. If the young man had known even a little bit of first aid, he might have been able to press the wound himself, and perhaps he wouldn't have died so young and far from home.

Let's Learn New First-Aid Skills

What to Do for Small Vessel Bleeding?

1. Direct Pressure to Stop the Bleeding
In simple terms, press where it's bleeding. This is the most commonly used, easiest to master, and quickest method in on-site first aid, typically used for bleeding from small arteries, small veins, or capillaries. It provides immediate hemostatic effect.

Things to Note:
When pressing the wound, avoid using your bare hands because human hands carry various bacteria that could cause infection. Additionally, direct contact between the hand and the wound may leave gaps, making the pressure less effective.

The Correct Approach:
First, place a sterile dressing on the wound, then apply pressure with your hand. If no sterile dressing is available at the scene, the best substitute is a clean piece of cloth. The easiest material to obtain is usually your own clothing.

Tear the clothing into strips, fold it several times to use as a dressing, place it over the wound, and press down firmly with your hand.

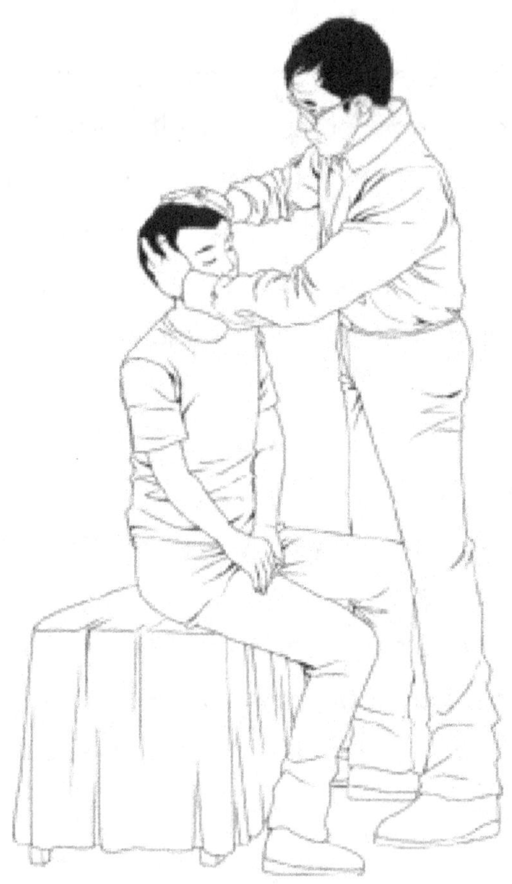

If the dressing becomes soaked with blood, should you quickly replace it with a new one? Absolutely not! This would be like repeatedly pressing a sponge against the wound to soak up the blood, which not only fails to stop the bleeding but can also increase the amount of blood loss. The correct approach is to place an additional dressing on top of the original one. In most cases, the bleeding can be controlled after applying pressure for a few minutes.

If the wound is on the upper limb, raise the limb above the level of the heart. If the wound is on the lower limb, have the injured person lie down and elevate the affected leg.

2. Compressive Bandaging to Stop Bleeding
After successfully stopping the bleeding with direct pressure, a compressive bandage should be applied. This involves layering the sterile dressing a bit thicker and wrapping it tightly enough to exert some pressure on the wound, helping to control further bleeding.

Note:
The bandage should not be too tight. If the limb becomes discolored (bluish-purple) or swollen after bandaging, it indicates that the bandage is too tight and may be affecting blood circulation. In such cases, the bandage should be loosened

and reapplied.

Situations Requiring the Packing Method for Bleeding Control

For cases involving bleeding from the nose, neck, armpit, groin, vagina, as well as non-penetrating wounds, penetrating injuries, deep wounds, or tissue loss, the packing method should be used. This involves filling the wound with sterile or clean fabric, packing it tightly, and then applying pressure with a bandage.

At the Scene of First Aid

A high school girl was climbing over the school fence with her friends when her foot slipped, and she ended up straddling a vertical fence post, which penetrated her vaginal area. When we arrived, her friends had already taken her down, but she was still bleeding and sitting on the ground, crying in agony.

We quickly lifted her onto the ambulance, and a

nurse used gauze soaked with liquid paraffin (for lubrication) to pack her vagina, stopping the bleeding. Afterward, we wrapped the area with a triangular bandage and rushed her to the hospital.

This was an extremely dangerous incident. Fortunately, the metal post that penetrated her vagina was not too long. If it had been longer and reached the abdominal cavity, it could have punctured the abdominal aorta, leading to unimaginable consequences.

Another time, late at night, we were called to a small hotel, where we found a large patch of fresh blood soaking through the sheets and mattress. We learned that it was a couple's first night together, and after intercourse, the woman experienced heavy bleeding. It didn't seem like the typical bleeding caused by a torn hymen, and the couple, terrified, called for an ambulance.

This was my first encounter with such a situation. I recalled my anatomy professor mentioning that rough intercourse could tear the posterior fornix of the vagina. Using gauze, I packed the woman's vagina tightly and applied a pressure bandage, which quickly stopped the bleeding.

We transported the patient to the gynecology department of Beijing Friendship Hospital, where a kind female doctor attended to her. I quietly asked the doctor, "Could you let me know the diagnosis afterward?"

A short while later, the doctor came out and confirmed, "You were right. It was indeed a tear of the posterior fornix."

Although such incidents are rare, I've since encountered three similar cases.

What about more common cases, like nosebleeds?

At the Scene of First Aid

Once, a friend from southern China came to Beijing on a business trip. We met for dinner, and he complained, "You can't live in Beijing! I washed my clothes last night, and they were already dry by the next morning. How can anyone live in such dry weather?"

He had spent most of his life in the humid south, and his nose couldn't tolerate Beijing's dry climate, which made his nasal membranes prone to bleeding. As he was speaking, his nose started bleeding again, and he immediately tilted his head back.

I quickly stopped him and asked him to tilt his head forward instead. Though he complied, he looked puzzled, so I explained the correct procedure to him.

Correct Nosebleed Management

When we were children, many parents and teachers told us to tilt our heads back when we had a nosebleed. However, this is incorrect.

Tilting the head back can cause blood to flow into the airway and lungs, potentially leading to suffocation. It may also cause the blood to enter the esophagus and digestive tract, which can irritate the stomach lining and trigger nausea or vomiting.

The correct way to stop a nosebleed is to lean slightly forward, lower the head, and breathe through the mouth. Use the thumb and index finger of one hand to pinch both nostrils and apply pressure upward and backward. In most cases, this method can stop the bleeding after a few minutes.

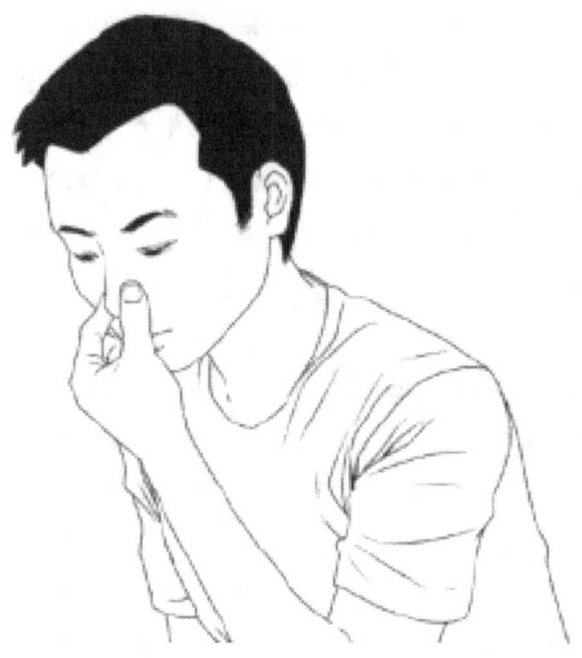

If the bleeding is caused by a blood disorder, nasopharyngeal cancer, hypertension, or nasal trauma, stopping the bleeding alone won't be enough—systemic treatment will also be required. In such cases, the patient should promptly go to the hospital. Additionally, the management of nosebleeds caused by a basilar skull fracture will be discussed in a later section.

The packing method can also be effective for both non-penetrating and penetrating injuries.

What Are "Non-penetrating" and "Penetrating" Injuries?

For example, with a stab wound, if the knife enters the body but doesn't exit—there's an entry wound but no exit wound—it is considered a *non-penetrating injury*. If the knife enters and exits, leaving both an entry and an exit wound, it is classified as a *penetrating injury*.

In both situations, sterile gauze can be used to pack the wound tightly and fully, followed by a pressure bandage. If sterile gauze isn't available, clean clothing can serve as a substitute.

Wound Bandaging: Learn to "Use What's Available"

Bandaging is one of the essential steps in first aid for external injuries. After effective bleeding control, the injured area should be promptly and correctly bandaged.

Why is learning how to bandage important? There are three key reasons:

1. For compressive bandaging to control bleeding.
2. To protect the wound from further injury or contamination.
3. To secure the dressing in place and relieve the patient's pain.

Once you master bandaging, you'll be able to handle minor injuries in daily life on your own.

Common Bandaging Methods

1. Circular Bandaging Method
This is the most basic bandaging technique. It is

suitable for areas such as the wrist, ankle, forehead, or other parts of the body with similar thickness. It is also used as the starting point for various other bandaging techniques.

To apply:
- Place the bandage slightly at an angle over the wound and wrap it around once.
- On the second wrap, fold the corner of the first layer that sticks out at an angle.
- Continue wrapping the third and fourth layers, pressing down on the folded corner to secure it.
- As you wrap, ensure each layer overlaps the previous one slightly.
- Finally, secure the end of the bandage with adhesive tape.

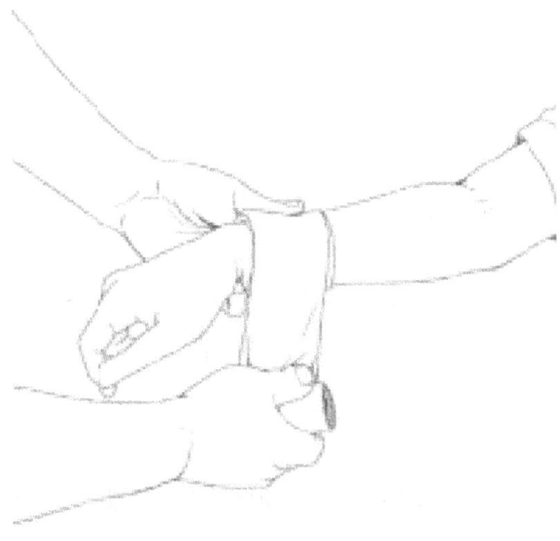

2. Spiral Bandaging Method

This method is mainly used for limbs or other areas with relatively uniform thickness.

How to Apply:

- Begin with two or three circular wraps following the circular bandaging method.

- Then, continue wrapping upward at an angle.

- Ensure that each layer overlaps the previous one by two-thirds.

- Secure the end of the bandage with adhesive tape.

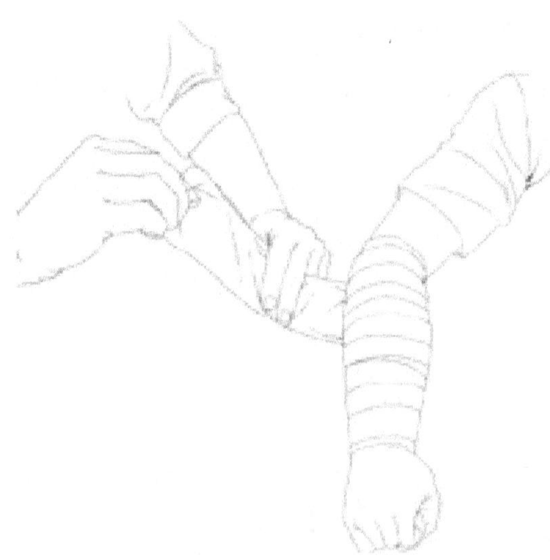

3.Reverse Spiral Bandaging Method

This method is used for bandaging areas with

uneven thickness, such as the forearm, lower leg, or thigh.

How to Apply:

1. Start with two circular wraps using the circular bandaging method.

2. Continue with the spiral bandaging method.

3. Press the center of the bandage with one hand's fingers, while using the other hand to fold the bandage downward.

4. Repeat the folding process as you continue wrapping.

5. Ensure that each fold is neatly aligned.

6. Be careful not to fold the bandage over the wound or on bony protrusions.

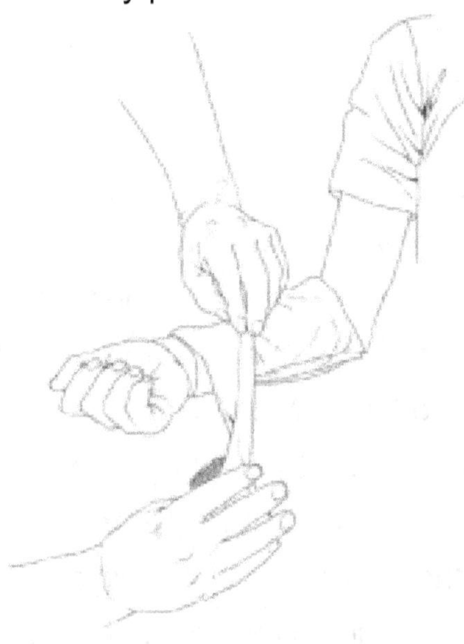

4.Figure-Eight Bandaging Method

This method is primarily used for bandaging the wrist, elbow, knee, foot, shoulder, and hip, as well as for immobilizing a clavicle fracture.

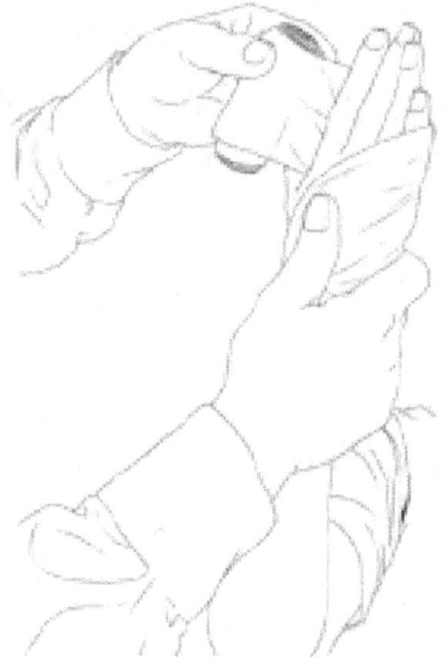

Using the elbow joint as an example, start by applying two circular wraps around the middle of the joint. Then, wrap the bandage from the bottom to the top around both sides of the joint, following the bend. Next, wrap it from the top to the bottom in a figure-eight pattern, repeating this back and forth. Ensure that each layer overlaps the previous one by two-thirds. Finally, finish with two circular wraps and secure the end with adhesive tape.

For other body parts, the method is similar, and you can apply the same principles without needing to provide specific examples for each one.

For bandaging an internal object, you can also use the figure-eight compression bandaging method. Before bandaging, place a roll of fabric on either side of the object.

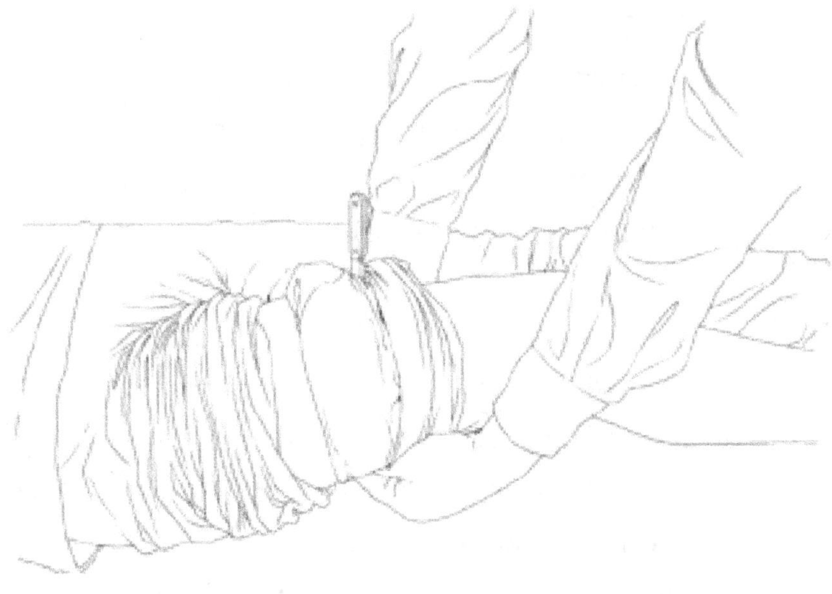

Return Bandaging Method
This method is suitable for bandaging the head

and residual limbs.

1. Start by applying two circular wraps around the area.
2. Then, repeatedly fold the bandage back and forth: the first fold is in the center, and each subsequent fold goes left and right until the wound is completely covered.
3. Finally, finish with two circular wraps.

Triangular Bandaging Method
The triangular bandaging method is the most commonly used, quickest, and most convenient technique in on-site first aid.

Hood-style Bandaging for the Head and Face:
The rescuer stands behind the injured person. Position the top corner of the triangular bandage along the midline of the back of the head. Fold the bottom edge inward about two finger widths and place it at the forehead, level with the eyebrows.

Then, pull the two bottom corners over the ears

towards the occipital region, crossing them below the occipital protuberance and pressing the top corner tightly. Wrap it back around the forehead and tie a knot. Finally, pull the top corner tight, fold it, and tuck it into the crossed area at the back of the head.

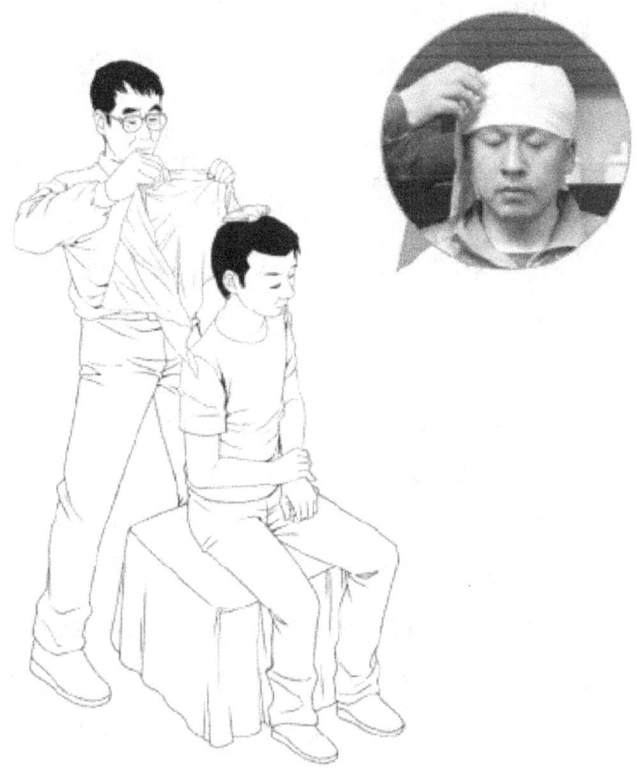

Mask-style Bandaging Method
The rescuer stands behind the injured person,

ties a knot at the top corner of the triangular bandage, and holds the two bottom edges. Then, tuck the top corner around the chin.

Next, pull the bottom edges towards the back of the head, lift the two bottom corners, and tighten them. Cross them at the back of the head, pressing the bottom edges tightly, and then wrap them around to the forehead to tie a knot.

After bandaging, lift the triangular bandage over the eyes, mouth, and nose, and cut small openings to expose the eyes and facial features.

Double Eye Bandaging Method
The rescuer stands behind the injured person and folds the triangular bandage into a strip about 3 to 4 finger widths wide. The midpoint is placed below the occipital region, with the two ends wrapped around from under the ears to cross over the eyes, covering both eyes. The ends are then pulled over the ears towards the back of the head and tied.

Shoulder Bandaging Method
The rescuer stands behind the injured person

and folds the triangular bandage into a swallowtail shape, ensuring the two swallowtail corners are of equal size, with an angle of approximately 120°. The angle should be directed upwards, aligned with the midline of the back of the neck. Each swallowtail should cover one shoulder, with the corners wrapping from front to back over the shoulder until they meet at the armpit and tie.

Chest (Back) Bandaging Method
The rescuer faces the injured person and folds the triangular bandage into a swallowtail shape, with the angle approximately 100°. Place the swallowtail bandage on the chest, aligning the angle with the suprasternal notch. Each swallowtail corner should cover the shoulders and extend to the back. The rescuer then moves to the back of the injured person and ties the top corner of the bandage with the bottom edge at the back. Pull the swallowtail corners tight, lifting them upward behind the horizontal bandage, and tie them together. (When bandaging the back, simply place the swallowtail bandage on the back; the rest of the steps are essentially the same as for chest bandaging.)

Unilateral Chest Bandaging Method

The rescuer faces the injured person and places the top corner of the triangular bandage on the injured side shoulder. The bottom edge is folded inward about two finger widths and wrapped around the chest to the back, where the two bottom corners meet and are tied. The rescuer moves to the back of the injured person, pulls the bottom corners towards the back, and ties them together.

Abdominal Bandaging Method

The rescuer faces the injured person and positions the bottom edge of the triangular bandage upwards, with the top corner facing down to cover the abdomen. The bottom edge should align with the waist, and the two bottom corners are tied at the back. The top corner is then pulled between the legs towards the back, where it is tied to the bottom corners.

Upper Limb Bandaging Method

Standing on the side of the injured limb, the rescuer ties one bottom corner of the triangular bandage and places it on the middle finger of the injured hand. The other bottom corner covers the same-side shoulder and back. The top corner is lifted upward, wrapping around the injured finger from outside to inside and securing it. Finally, bend the forearm across the chest, placing the hand on the healthy side's clavicle, and tie the two bottom corners together.

Lower Leg and Foot Bandaging Method
With the toes facing the bottom edge, position the foot on the side of one bottom corner. Lift the top corner and wrap it with the other bottom corner around the lower leg, tying it. Then, fold the lower corner of the foot over the dorsum and tie it around the ankle.

Important Note: If there is protrusion of brain tissue from a wound or the intestine and greater omentum protrude, do not apply pressure to bandage. First, cover the area with a large piece of disinfected, moist gauze, then use rolled gauze to create a protective ring around the protruding brain tissue or intestine and greater omentum. Finally, place an appropriately sized bowl, basin, or similar vessel over the ring and secure it with a triangular bandage to avoid compressing the brain tissue.

Making a Suspended Arm Sling

Large Suspended Arm Sling: This method is primarily used for injuries to the forearm or elbow joint and is prohibited for humeral fractures.

Place one bottom corner of the triangular bandage on the shoulder of the healthy side, ensuring the bottom edge is parallel to the body's longitudinal axis. The top corner should face the elbow of the injured side, with the elbow slightly flexed at less than 90° (the hand should be higher than the elbow) placed in the middle of the triangular bandage. The other bottom corner is folded back and wrapped around the forearm, passing through the shoulder of the injured side. The two bottom corners are tied at the back of the neck, allowing the forearm to hang in front of the chest.

Small Suspended Arm Sling

This method is primarily used for injuries to the upper arm or shoulder joint.

1. Fold the triangular bandage into a strip of appropriate width.

2. Position the center of the strip at the lower third of the forearm on the injured side.

3. Bring the two bottom corners over the shoulders and tie them at the back of the neck, allowing the forearm to hang in front of the chest with the hand slightly higher than the elbow.

4. The elbow joint should be flexed at an angle of approximately 80° to 85°.

5. Use a restraining band to secure it in place, preventing movement of the shoulder joint.

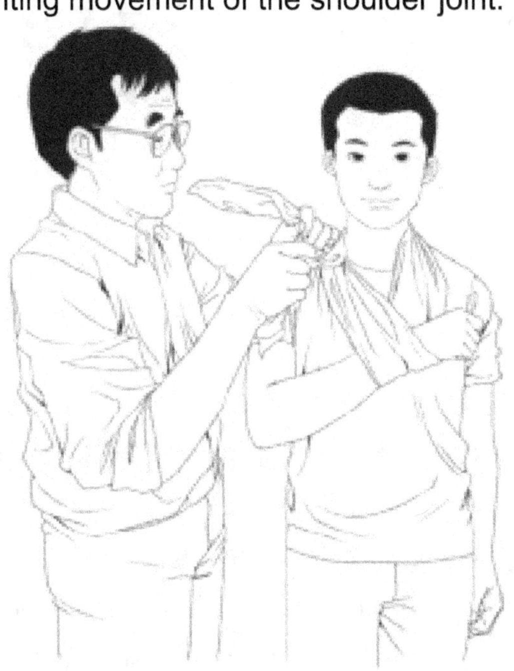

Triangular Suspended Arm Sling

This method can be used for bandaging, immobilizing, and suspending injuries to the clavicle, elbow joint, forearm, and hand.

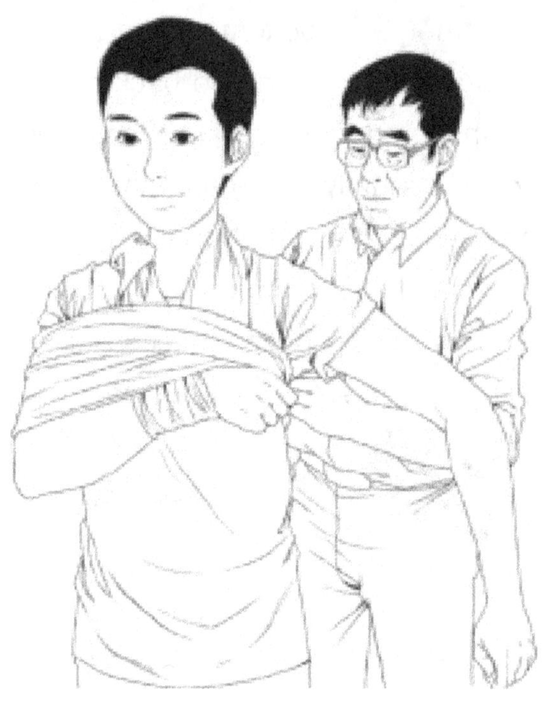

Instruct the injured person to bring their five fingers together, placing the middle finger on the supraclavicular notch of the opposite shoulder. Facing the injured person, hold the top corner and one bottom corner of the triangular bandage with both hands. The top corner should cover the elbow on the injured side, while the bottom corner is pulled towards the opposite shoulder to cover the hand. At this point, the triangular bandage will have covered the entire hand and forearm.

Next, fold the triangular bandage below the forearm to the back of the arm. Then, rotate the top corner along with the bottom edge several times. Tie the two bottom corners together where they meet at the opposite shoulder. A restraining band can also be used as needed.

What to Do When Clean Materials Are Unavailable

Since emergencies can occur in various situations, what should you do if you cannot find sterile gauze or a triangular bandage? It's not just ordinary people; even professional doctors may encounter unexpected situations without sterile gauze on hand. In fact, any clean fabric can be used; as mentioned earlier, clean clothing, bed sheets, curtains, towels, scarves, etc., can all work. You can improvise based on the situation and tear them as needed.

In on-site first aid, the most commonly used, quickest, and most convenient bandaging material is the military triangular bandage. This was invented by Israeli soldiers, featuring a canvas exterior with two plastic pieces inside, making it waterproof, moisture-resistant, and sterile. Triangular bandages are available at pharmacies, and they can also be homemade. For families with cars, it is advisable to keep them in a vehicle's first aid kit.

Additionally, when using a bandage, the wrapping technique should depend on the specific situation. For example, use the circular bandaging method for areas with similar thickness. If there is a hole at the wound site, you'll need to use the spiral bandaging method. If that isn't effective, you can switch to the reverse spiral bandaging method.

After bandaging, be sure to tie it off; usually, a piece of adhesive tape will suffice. Of course, special areas such as a woman's nipples or a man's external genitalia should be avoided, and the bandage should be tightened appropriately.

If it is a limb injury, try to leave the distal end exposed for the doctor to observe later.

Burn Injury Treatment: Three Steps - Rinse, Cover, and Go

Burns refer to specific injuries caused by various heat sources (flames, hot water, hot oil, steam, gasoline, strong acids, alkalis, quicklime, phosphorus, electrical burns, etc.). People often refer to injuries from hot liquids as scalds, but these are also considered burns.

Burns are a common accidental injury, especially during July and August when the weather is hot, and people wear lighter clothing, making them more susceptible to burns from hot water, oil, porridge, etc. As a result, burn units in hospitals become particularly busy during the summer. Many people panic when faced with burns and don't know how to respond; improper treatment can easily lead to adverse outcomes.

I often see cases where parents rush their child to the hospital without any first aid after the child is scalded by hot water. This usually takes at least ten minutes, and sometimes, due to intense pain, the child might tear off the burnt skin. In fact, after a burn occurs, the first thing to do is to quickly escape the danger and initiate immediate first aid to minimize damage. Home self-rescue often helps reduce the severity of the injury and aids recovery.

More than 80% of the damage caused by burns is due to residual heat, so the key to first aid is to minimize this residual heat. Rinsing with cool water is the most effective way to reduce the damage from residual heat. Rinse or soak the wound in cool water (15-25°C) for about 20 minutes to neutralize the residual heat, lower the temperature, relieve pain, reduce damage, and prevent scar formation. Avoid using ice; this is a common misconception. Applying ice to freshly burned skin causes excessive blood vessel constriction, which hinders recovery.

For burns from strong acids, alkalis, or quicklime, it is even more critical to rinse thoroughly with plenty of water for 20-30 minutes. Some may wonder, "Didn't my teacher say in middle school that you shouldn't pour water on sulfuric acid because it generates more heat?"

If burned by sulfuric acid, you should first wipe it off with a cloth to minimize the amount left on the skin, and then rinse thoroughly with a large volume of water to prevent the burn area from expanding.

Wet clothing should be removed under cold water. If it sticks to the skin, do not forcibly tear it off. Instead, cut around the wound and remove watches, bracelets, rings, etc., to avoid circulation issues caused by swelling. If blisters form, do not pop them to avoid infection. After treating the burn locally, cover the wound with a sterile or clean cloth, then go to the hospital as quickly as possible.

Remember, do not apply any substances to the wound, especially toothpaste, soy sauce, soybean paste, baking soda, or plant ash. These not only fail to treat the burn but may also lead to infections, which can be dangerous.

Many people ask if burns should be bandaged. My suggestion is both yes and no. Why? Bandages might stick to the wound and cause skin damage when removed at the hospital. However, if left uncovered, exposure to the air can lead to infection. In severe burns, infection is the main cause of death in the later stages.

So, what should be done? Use a clean cloth to cover the burn and head to the hospital quickly. Upon arrival, removing the cloth should not cause significant problems.

In conclusion, the three critical steps for burn treatment are: rinse, cover, and go. Nothing more.

Key Points for Burn Treatment:

1. For minor burns, rinse with cool running water (such as tap water) for 20-30 minutes until the pain subsides. For burns caused by strong acids, alkalis, or quicklime, wipe with a cloth first and then rinse thoroughly with water for 20-30 minutes.
2. For severe burns, follow the three-step principle:
    - Rinse: Quickly rinse the wound with cool

water (15-25°C) for 20 minutes.

- Cover: Cover the wound with a clean cloth.

- Go: Proceed to the hospital for professional treatment.

3. Important Reminders:

- Do not use ice packs, puncture blisters, or apply ointments.

- Cut off clothing stuck to the wound without pulling it away.

Severe Trauma: Do Not Rinse or Apply Medications Indiscriminately

Earlier, we discussed how burns should be promptly rinsed with cool water. However, does this approach apply to other types of wounds? The answer is no, and indiscriminate use of medications on wounds should also be avoided. Here's why:

Many sources suggest that wounds should first be rinsed with clean water, but this is not entirely correct. For minor injuries, such as a scraped or punctured skin, gently rinsing with clean water and applying a bit of medication is usually fine. In these cases, hospital treatment might not even be necessary, as minor wounds tend to heal quickly on their own.

However, when it comes to severe wounds, rinsing with water can push contaminants deeper into the wound, increasing the risk of infection.

For significant bleeding, especially when a major blood vessel is ruptured, stopping the bleeding relies primarily on applying pressure. Small blood vessels often rely on natural clotting, where microthrombi (tiny blood clots) form to plug the bleeding site. If clots form in intact blood vessels, they can cause serious conditions like acute heart attacks or strokes. But when they form at a damaged blood vessel, it serves as a protective mechanism to stop bleeding. Rinsing with water dilutes the blood, interfering with coagulation and hampering the body's natural ability to stop the bleeding.

While it's important to adhere to medical principles, practical situations may require flexibility.

Real-life Emergency Response Example:

About 30 years ago, in the early hours of a summer morning at a construction site near Beijing's Match Factory, a worker's leg was completely severed by a winch. Fellow workers immediately called for emergency help.

When we arrived at the scene, it was dark, and we saw the injured man lying on the ground, unconscious, with his severed leg nearby. He was pale, and his body was covered in sand and cement slurry. The mixture of blood and cement on the wound made it impossible to see clearly.

I used a water hose nearby, which was still running, to rinse off the cement slurry from the wound. This did not involve pushing contaminants deeper into the wound but rather allowed us to see the bleeding vessels clearly. I quickly clamped the blood vessels with hemostats to control the bleeding and wrapped them along with the clamps.

The workers told me that the bleeding had been severe, spraying blood everywhere, even on their clothes and faces. This showed that the most critical bleeding phase had passed, and the bleeding had somewhat subsided by the time we arrived.

While listening to the workers' account, I continued to treat the patient. I checked his blood pressure, which was zero. I immediately established two intravenous lines and rapidly administered blood plasma substitute and saline. After stabilizing his condition, we quickly transported him to Peking Union Medical College Hospital.

Why You Shouldn't Apply Medications to Severe Wounds:

Apart from avoiding water rinsing for severe wounds, applying topical medications without guidance is also inadvisable. When the patient reaches the hospital, the medical team will need to reconnect nerves, arteries, veins, tendons, and muscles accurately. If you've applied medications like red or purple antiseptics, the wound may be stained, making it harder for doctors to identify and suture the different tissues correctly. This will complicate and delay medical treatment.

In summary, whether it's rinsing with water or applying ointments, these actions can hinder the doctor's ability to treat the wound effectively.

Therefore, it's essential not to try to help in ways that may cause more harm, avoiding what is often described as "good intentions gone wrong."

Sprained Ankles and Severed Limbs: Returning Everything to Its Place

One common issue people ask about is ankle sprains, also known as "twisted ankles." Whether in daily life, work, travel, or sports, walking, running, and jumping are inevitable activities. On uneven surfaces, stairs, or slopes, it's easy to twist an ankle, especially for women wearing high heels or thick-soled shoes.

The ankle joint is complex, with weak muscles and poor protection, but it bears a significant load. When standing, your entire body weight presses down on the ankles, and when taking a step, all your weight shifts onto one ankle. Most ankle sprains involve the foot rolling inward, injuring the lateral ligaments. Depending on the severity, this can range from partial tears to complete ruptures, often accompanied by bruising and swelling.

I once visited the Xicheng District Planning Commission in Beijing and saw an injured man sitting on the ground, surrounded by his colleagues. He had injured himself while walking on flat ground, and his bone was protruding. This was no longer just a sprain but a fracture. While sprained ankles are common, such severe cases are rare.

Apart from sprained ankles, we also need to talk about severed limbs. Although this may seem distant from most people's lives, I once encountered a case where a man impulsively cut off his own finger.

Sprained Ankle First Aid:

1. Stop Movement: Have the injured person stop walking or moving, and immediately take a seated or lying position, raising the limb to promote venous return.
2. Cold Compress: Apply an ice pack or cool towel to the affected area. This helps constrict blood vessels, reducing leakage and swelling. During the first 48 hours after the injury, apply

cold compresses every 2-3 hours for 15-20 minutes at a time.

3. Avoid Movement After Cooling: Keep the foot in a position with the outer side elevated and the inner side lowered. Use a wide adhesive bandage, triangular scarf, or bandage to immobilize the area. If there's a fracture, follow fracture immobilization guidelines and head to the hospital immediately.

Important Note: Do not massage the injured area, and avoid using hot compresses within the first 24 hours. Heat can cause blood vessels to dilate, increasing fluid leakage and swelling. Hot compresses should only be used 24-48 hours after the injury.

Real-life Emergency Example:

In one incident, a young couple was arguing because the girl wanted to break up. The boy, after pleading with her unsuccessfully, impulsively grabbed a kitchen knife and cut off his little finger in front of her. The girl was terrified and immediately called for an ambulance. When I arrived, I asked where the severed finger was, and the boy spat it out from his mouth. I quickly had him wrap it in cloth, place it in a plastic bag, and then put that bag into another bag containing ice. This process is called cold preservation, which lowers the metabolic rate and oxygen consumption of the severed finger, buying more time and better conditions for reattachment.

Over the years, I've encountered many cases of severed fingers and limbs. Usually, as long as reattachment is done within a certain timeframe (generally 6-8 hours), the severed limb can be successfully reattached.

I asked the boy why he kept the severed finger in his mouth, and he explained that he feared other places might not be clean. Thinking about it, he decided not to put it in his pocket, so he kept it in his mouth. However, the mouth contains many bacteria and is not necessarily cleaner than a pocket. Moreover, the mouth's high temperature and digestive enzymes could slowly begin to break down the severed tissue.

On another occasion, a young patient was brought to the emergency center by a doctor wearing a white coat, who had come from a local clinic. The doctor took a bottle from his pocket containing the severed finger and said, "Just attach it on the operating table; I've already disinfected it!"

Dr. Sun, our surgeon, asked him, "What did you use to disinfect it?"

"Alcohol," the young doctor replied.

Dr. Sun immediately lost his temper. "Are you even a doctor?"

The young doctor was stunned and said, "Yes, I work in our factory's clinic."

"If you're a doctor, don't you understand what alcohol is for?"

"For disinfection," he replied.

"And how does it disinfect?"

"By coagulating bacterial proteins."

"Did it ever occur to you that it also coagulates normal tissue proteins?"

At that moment, the young doctor realized his mistake, but by then, the improper handling meant the finger was no longer viable for reattachment.

First Aid for Severed Limbs:
1. Stop the Bleeding and Bandage the Wound: After controlling the bleeding, tend to the severed limb.
2. Do Not Rinse the Severed Limb: No matter how dirty it is, do not wash it. Keep it dry by wrapping it in a clean cloth or towel. Place it in a plastic bag and tie it securely.
3. Store on Ice: Find another plastic bag, place ice inside, and then put the bag containing the severed limb into the ice bag. If ice is unavailable, frozen items like ice cream bars or frozen meat from the freezer can be used.

Why Use Ice? Cold temperatures lower the metabolic rate and oxygen consumption of the severed limb, allowing it to tolerate a longer period without blood supply. This buys time for successful reattachment.

Why Use Two Layers of Plastic Bags? The outer bag provides a cold environment, while the inner bag prevents the severed limb from direct contact with water. If the severed tissue swells and ruptures after soaking, reattachment becomes impossible. Why wrap it in cloth before placing it on ice? Direct contact with ice can cause the temperature to drop too low, leading to excessive blood vessel constriction and difficulty during the rewarming process.

By understanding these critical emergency responses, you can significantly increase the chances of successful recovery and reattachment for injuries like sprains and severed limbs.

Fracture Immobilization: The Key is "Stabilization"

When dealing with falls or other injuries, determining whether the person has a fracture is crucial. Once a fracture is confirmed, it should be immobilized immediately. For the general public, it can sometimes be challenging to distinguish between a dislocation and a fracture, so it's advisable to treat it as a fracture for immobilization purposes. Common fractures such as those in the limbs or ribs can usually be identified by observation and simple touch. However, for certain areas, even a professional emergency doctor like myself might occasionally overlook a fracture.

There are many types of fractures, with the most common being open and closed fractures. Simply put, an open fracture occurs when the bone breaks and pierces through the skin, making the bone visible from the outside. A closed fracture involves a broken bone without any skin wound.

Typically, an open fracture requires bleeding to be controlled first, followed by immobilization. It is important to note that the goal is "immobilization," not "realignment" or "correcting deformities." The purpose of immobilization is to "stabilize" the limb, limiting its movement. For example, if the femur is fractured and no treatment is given before transporting the patient to the hospital, the sharp edges of the broken bone could potentially damage surrounding nerves during transit, worsening the injury.

Different parts of the body require specific methods for immobilization. Below are several techniques for immobilizing fractures in different areas, which can often be used interchangeably.

Upper Arm Fracture Immobilization
Splint Method: Place two splints on the inner and outer sides of the upper arm (if only one splint is available, place it on the outer side of the upper arm). Use bandages or a triangular bandage to secure both ends of the splints. Then, suspend the forearm in front of the chest with a small sling, allowing the elbow joint to bend. Use a

folded strap across the upper part of the forearm, connecting it with the small sling and securing the upper arm to the torso, which helps to restrict shoulder joint movement.

Torso Method: If no splint is available, a triangular bandage can be folded into a strip 10–15 cm wide, with its center placed directly over the fracture site to secure the upper arm to the torso. Then, suspend the forearm in front of the chest with a small sling, allowing the elbow joint to bend.

Forearm Fracture Immobilization

Splint Method: Place two splints, running from the elbow to the palm, on the palmar (palm) and dorsal (back) sides of the forearm (if only one splint is available, place it on the dorsal side). Cushion the palm with cotton or other soft material, and have the patient grip the splint, with the wrist slightly bent towards the palm. Secure both ends of the splints, and then use a larger sling to suspend the forearm in front of the chest, allowing the elbow joint to bend.

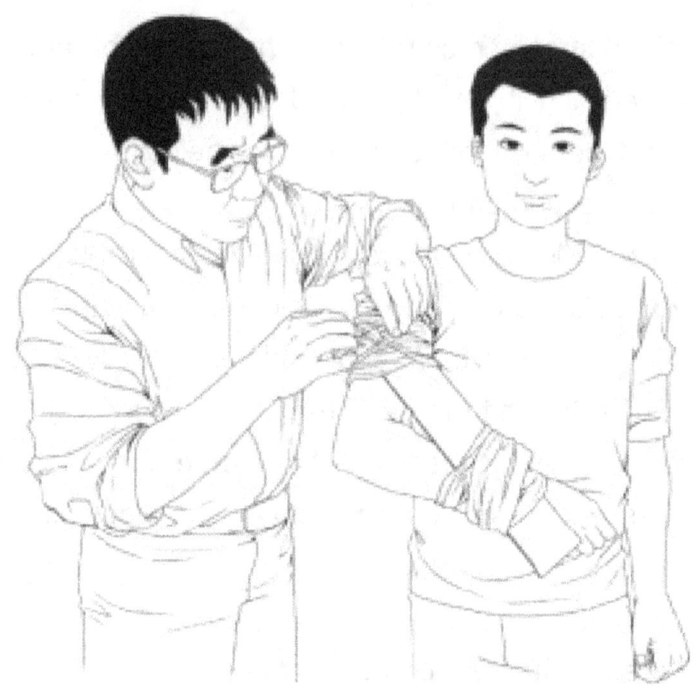

Garment and Torso Immobilization Method:

When no splint is available, the patient's own clothing can be used for immobilization. Bend the injured side's elbow so that the forearm rests against the chest, and tuck the hand into the space between the third and fourth buttons of the shirt. Then, fold the injured side's garment flap outward, lift it, and turn it up, fastening the buttons on the injured side's flap with the buttonholes on the healthy side's flap (alternatively, use a strap to tie the lower corner of the injured side's garment flap to the collar of the healthy side). Finally, use a belt or a strip of triangular bandage to wrap around the area just above the injured side's elbow and tie it securely, ensuring that the movement of both the upper arm and forearm is restricted.

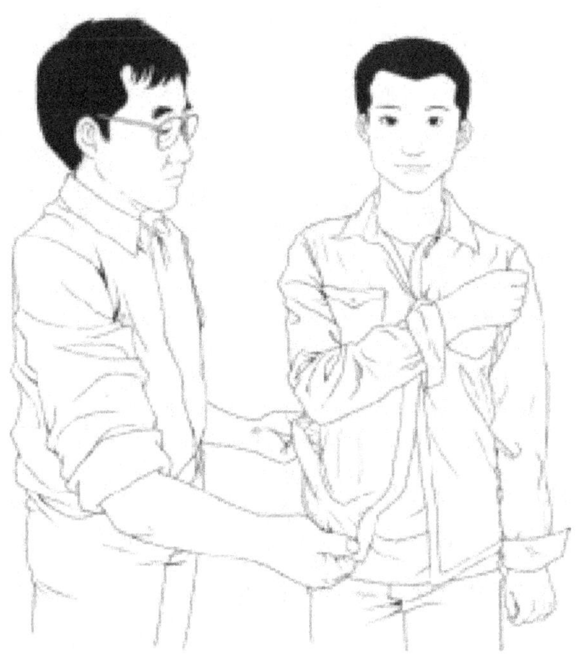

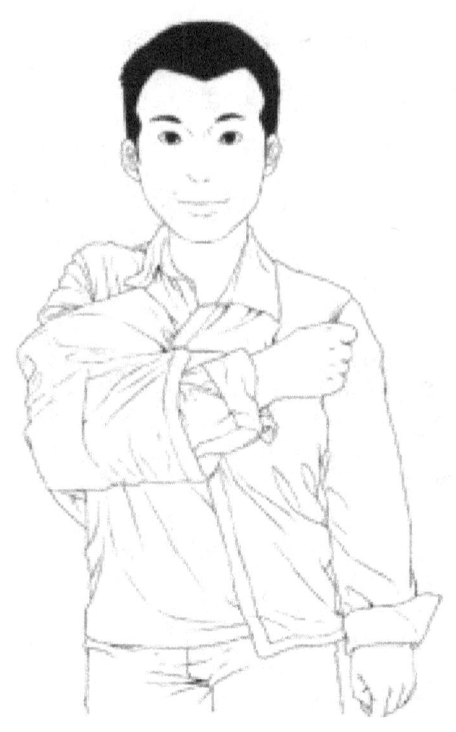

Thigh Fracture Immobilization

Splint Method: Have the patient lie on their back with the injured leg straightened. Place two splints along the inner and outer sides of the thigh. The outer splint should extend from the armpit to the heel, while the inner splint should run from the upper thigh to the heel (if only one splint is available, place it on the outer side of the thigh, using the healthy leg as the inner splint). Add padding at the joints and any gaps. Then, use cloth straps to secure the upper and lower ends of the fracture site, and further secure the chest, waist, knee, and ankle areas. The ankle and foot should be fixed in a figure-8 pattern to prevent the injured foot from rotating outward.

Healthy Limb Immobilization Method: When no splint is available, use cloth straps to bind the injured limb to the healthy limb. Add padding between the knees and ankles. First, secure the upper and lower ends of the fracture site, then secure above the knee joint and around the ankle joint. The ankle and foot should be fixed in a figure-8 pattern (refer to the "Splint Method").

For finger fractures, if a splint is not available, the injured finger can be immobilized by securing it to a healthy finger. Items like pencils, pens, or small sticks can be used as substitutes for a splint.

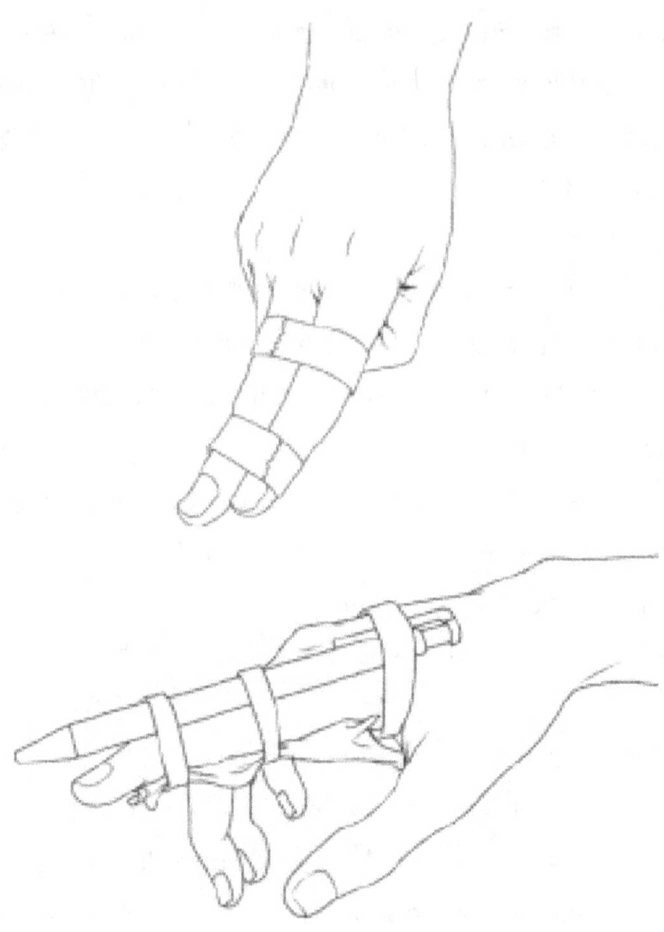

Thigh Fracture, Tying Sequence:

1. Ankle joint and foot

2. Below the knee joint

3. Upper end near the fracture site

4. Lower end near the fracture site

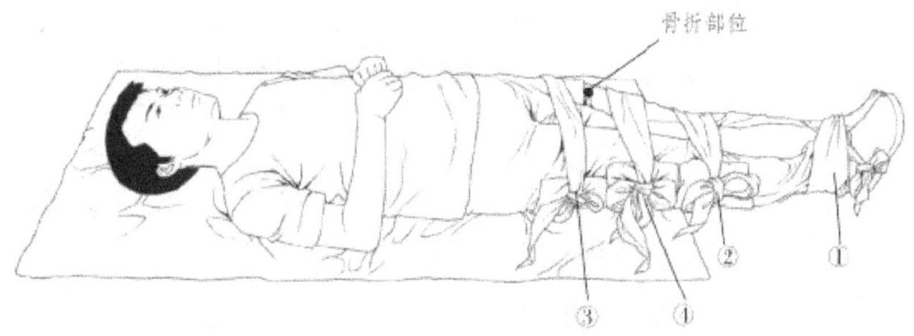

Lower Leg Fracture Immobilization

Splint Method: Place two splints, running from the lower thigh to the heel, along the inner and outer sides of the lower leg (if only one splint is available, place it on the outer side of the lower leg, using the healthy leg as the inner splint). Add padding around the joints, then secure the upper and lower ends of the fracture site first, followed by the middle of the thigh, knee, and ankle. The ankle and foot should be fixed in a figure-8 pattern (refer to "Thigh Fracture Immobilization").

Healthy Limb Immobilization Method: If no splint is available, use cloth straps to bind the injured leg to the healthy leg. Add padding between the knees and ankles. First, secure the upper and lower ends of the fracture site, then secure above the knee joint and around the ankle joint. The ankle and foot should be fixed in a figure-8 pattern (refer to "Splint Method").

Lower Leg Fracture, Tying Sequence:
1. Ankle joint and foot
2. Middle of the thigh
3. Upper end near the fracture site
4. Lower end near the fracture site

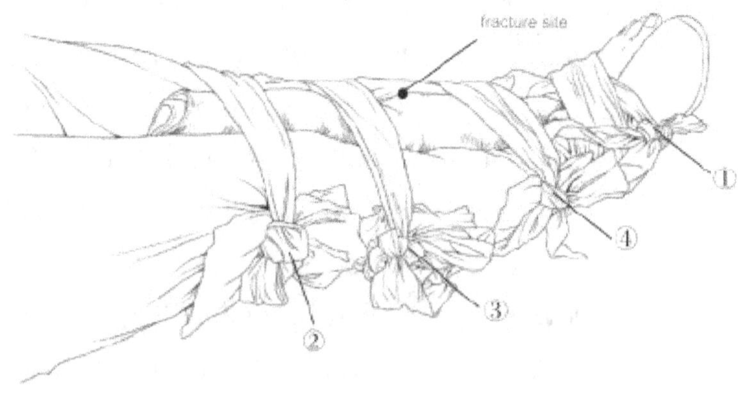

Mandibular (Jaw) Fracture

Fold a strap to a width of about one palm. Place the strap at the 1/3 and 2/3 junction under the patient's chin, cradling both sides of the jaw and covering the ears. The longer end should pass over the top of the head, cross over the opposite ear, then pass across the forehead just above the eyebrows. The ends of the strap should meet on the opposite side and be tied securely.

Clavicle (Collarbone) Fracture

Use two straps, securing each on either shoulder. Connect the ends of the straps behind the back and tie them, slightly pulling the patient's shoulders backward and pushing the chest forward. Alternatively, place padding under both armpits, and use a folded strap in a horizontal figure-8 around the shoulders, pulling the shoulders back and pushing the chest forward. Cross and tie the strap at the back to secure.

Rib Fracture

Rib fractures commonly occur between the 4th and 7th ribs. Use three straps folded to a width of four to five fingers, and wrap them around the chest, tightening after exhaling. Tie the straps at the opposite side of the body along the midline, ensuring consistent tension across all three straps.

Pelvic Fracture

First, stabilize the hips, then place padding

between the knees. Use a strap to bind the knees together.

What to Use When No Splint is Available

If no splint is at hand, many household items can be used, such as blankets or pillows. Fold a blanket thickly and place it around the fracture, then secure it with a bandage. If using a pillow, check the filling; pillows filled with buckwheat husks, common in the north, tend to shift and are not suitable for immobilization. Cotton-filled pillows, on the other hand, can be used to fully encase the injured area.

Additionally, a hard board can be placed around the fracture. If no wooden board or cardboard is available, newspapers or magazines can also be used. I once performed on-site emergency care for an elderly woman with a fracture using only newspapers for immobilization.

Over the years, I have often used magazines and newspapers for fracture immobilization in emergency situations. These materials are sometimes even more effective than professional equipment—easy to find, inexpensive, and soft enough not to cause abrasions like a hard board might.

On-site fracture care is not particularly difficult. The most important thing is to genuinely restrict movement of the injured area, preventing further damage caused by movement.

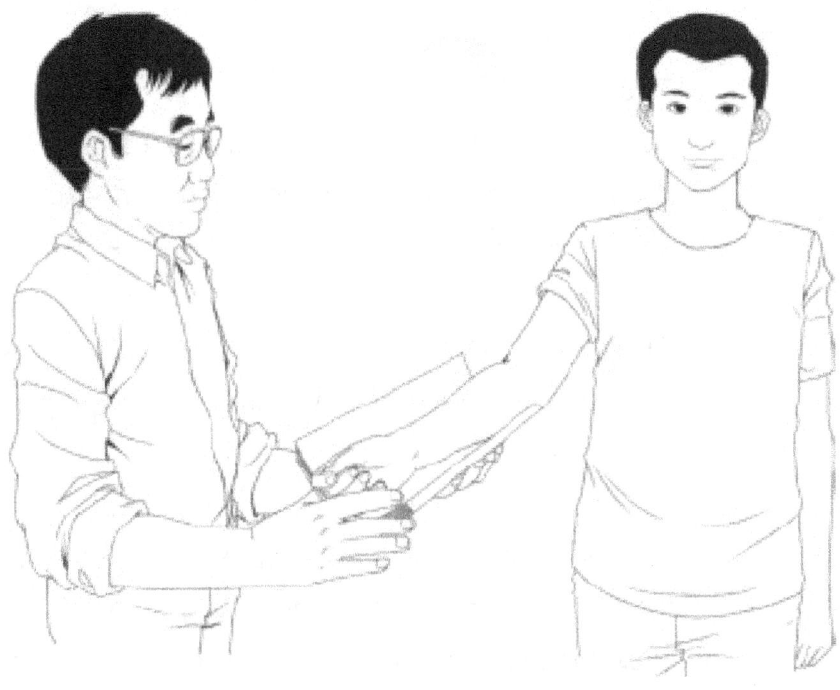

I would like to highlight basilar skull fractures.
Do you know where the base of the skull is?
The bones of the head are called the cranial bones, which encase the brain. The bones that

cover the top of the brain are known as the cranial vault, while those that support the brain are called the cranial base. The cranial base is located deep within the head and generally does not fracture easily. However, if a person is involved in a car accident or falls from a significant height, the cranial base may sustain a fracture due to the massive impact.

The cranial base is situated at the center of the head, and unlike limb fractures, it cannot be directly observed. However, there are some reliable indirect signs that can indicate a basilar skull fracture.

Fractures in different parts of the cranial base manifest in different ways. For example, periorbital hematoma, also known as the "raccoon eye sign," and mastoid hematoma (swelling behind the ears) are potential indicators. Additionally, there may be epistaxis (nosebleeds), which should be distinguished from those caused by nasal dryness, trauma, nasopharyngeal carcinoma, blood disorders, hypertension, etc., as well as otorrhea (bleeding from the ear), also referred to as "nasal leakage" or "ear leakage." When such symptoms appear, one should consider the possibility of a basilar skull fracture.

If there is a suspected basilar skull fracture, and symptoms like "nasal leakage" or "ear leakage" are present, what should you do?

1. Do not attempt to stop the bleeding. Not only should compression, packing, or rinsing to stop the bleeding be strictly prohibited, but the blood should also be allowed to flow out naturally. Position the patient so the injured side is down, allowing for full drainage. If blood is coming from an ear, turn that ear downward; if there is a nosebleed, tilt the head forward.

Why should you not compress the area to stop the bleeding? The source of the bleeding is at the cranial base, not the nose. Pressing the nose will not stop the bleeding from the cranial base, and it will prevent blood from flowing out through the nasal cavity. If the blood cannot drain, intracranial pressure will increase. Elevated intracranial pressure can compress the brain tissue, which is extremely dangerous.

Additionally, if the nose is pinched to stop bleeding, the blood can flow back into the nasal cavity, which is quite unhygienic. If the contaminated blood reverses back into the cranial cavity, it can lead to a brain infection, which can be life-threatening.

2. Keep the mouth clean and instruct the patient not to blow their nose.

This is to prevent increased intracranial pressure and the risk of intracranial infection. Also, call emergency services (dial 120) promptly to take the patient to a hospital for further diagnosis and treatment.

Let's Learn New First-Aid Skills
Key Points for Fracture Immobilization
1. Life first, then injury treatment. If the patient has no heartbeat or is not breathing, perform CPR immediately. If there is bleeding from a major vessel, apply effective measures to stop the bleeding.
2. For open fractures, control the bleeding first, then apply a bandage, and immobilize. For closed fractures, proceed directly to immobilization. If the lower limb is fractured,

immobilize it on the spot.

3. When using a splint, it must support the entire injured limb. The splint should not directly touch the skin; always place soft padding between the splint and the skin.

4. Do not attempt to push the broken ends of a bone back into the wound; do not attempt to realign the bone.

5. When immobilizing limb fractures, secure the proximal end first, followed by the distal end, without reversing the order. Also, try to expose the distal ends of the limbs.

6. For fractures of the humerus, ulna, or radius, bend the elbow joint slightly less than 90° and use a sling to suspend the arm in front of the chest. For fractures of the femur, tibia, or fibula, keep the knee joint straight.

Transporting the Injured: Be Careful, Extra Careful

For critically injured patients, once emergency first aid on site stabilizes them for transport, they need to be safely and quickly transported to a hospital for further treatment. Proper handling during transport is essential; if done incorrectly, it can undo all prior efforts, potentially resulting in lifelong disability or even death. Therefore, mastering correct transport techniques is a key skill for any rescuer.

Often, for patients with relatively minor injuries, we need to carry them to the hospital. Carrying an injured person is not just about physical strength—it requires technique, especially when the patient may weigh more than the rescuer. Below, I will introduce some common methods of transporting injured individuals.

Let's Learn New First-Aid Skills
Situations Suitable for Various Methods of Transporting the Injured
1. Assisted Walking: Suitable for patients with

minor injuries, without lower limb fractures, and able to walk on their own.

2. Carrying Method: Not recommended for patients with spinal injuries or lower limb fractures.

3. Piggyback Method: Not suitable for patients with spinal or limb fractures.

4. Dragging Method: Suitable for individuals who are heavier in weight.

5. Crawling Method: Suitable for patients with acute carbon monoxide (gas) poisoning.

6. Chair Carry or Stretcher Carry: These methods are suitable for conscious but physically weak patients.

7. Two-Person Cart Style Carry: Suitable for unconscious patients; not recommended for those with spinal or limb fractures.

Additionally, do not attempt to move a person with a spinal injury unless absolutely necessary.

Assisted Walking

This method is suitable for patients with minor injuries, no lower limb fractures, and who can walk on their own.

If there is only one rescuer nearby, they can

stand to one side of the patient, placing the patient's closest arm over the rescuer's shoulder, and hold it. The rescuer's other hand should reach around the patient's back, firmly supporting their armpit or waist, and they can walk together. If there are two rescuers, they should position themselves on either side of the patient, placing each of the patient's arms over their shoulders, and cross-support the patient's armpits or waist as they walk.

Carrying Method

The rescuer places one arm behind the patient's back, supporting their armpit, and the other arm under the patient's thighs, then lifts the patient up. Note that this method is not suitable for patients with spinal injuries or lower limb fractures.

Piggyback Method

The rescuer squats down, allowing the patient to lie on their back, and grasps the patient's wrists or uses their hands to secure the patient's thighs before slowly standing up. Alternatively, the rescuer can secure one of the patient's hands, insert the other arm between the patient's legs, and have the patient lie over their shoulder, slowly standing up while securing one of the patient's legs. This method is not suitable for those with spinal or limb fractures.

Dragging Method
This method is useful for transporting heavier individuals.
Place your hands under the patient's armpits or hold their ankles, and drag them. Alternatively, you can loosen the shirt of a supine patient, pull it over their head, and drag them by the collar. Using blankets or quilts can also be effective.

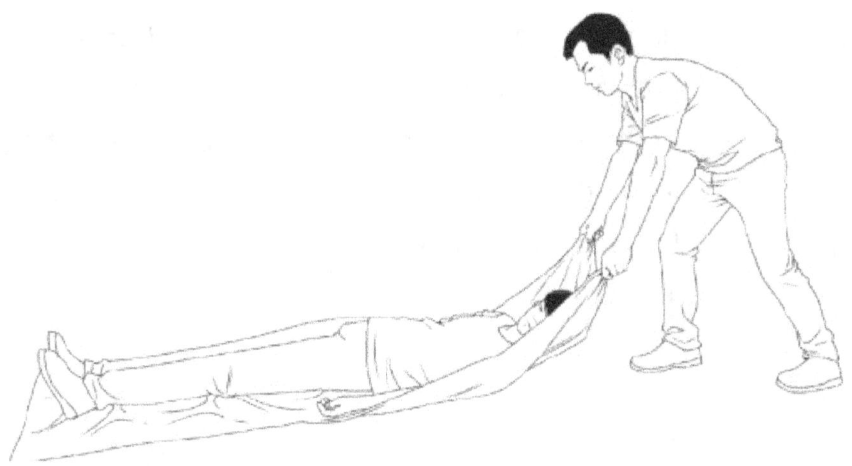

Crawling Method
This method is suitable for patients with acute

carbon monoxide (gas) poisoning.

Place the patient in a supine position, and use a towel, tie, or similar item to secure their wrists together. Straddle the patient with their hands secured around your neck, and use your hands to crawl, guiding the patient safely away from the scene.

Chair Carry Method

This method is suitable for conscious but physically weak patients.

Two rescuers position themselves on either side of the patient, facing each other. Each rescuer places one hand behind the patient's back, gripping their belt, and the other hand under the patient's thigh, grasping the other rescuer's wrist. Then, both rescuers slowly stand up, stepping forward with their outer leg first, and walk in sync to transport the patient.

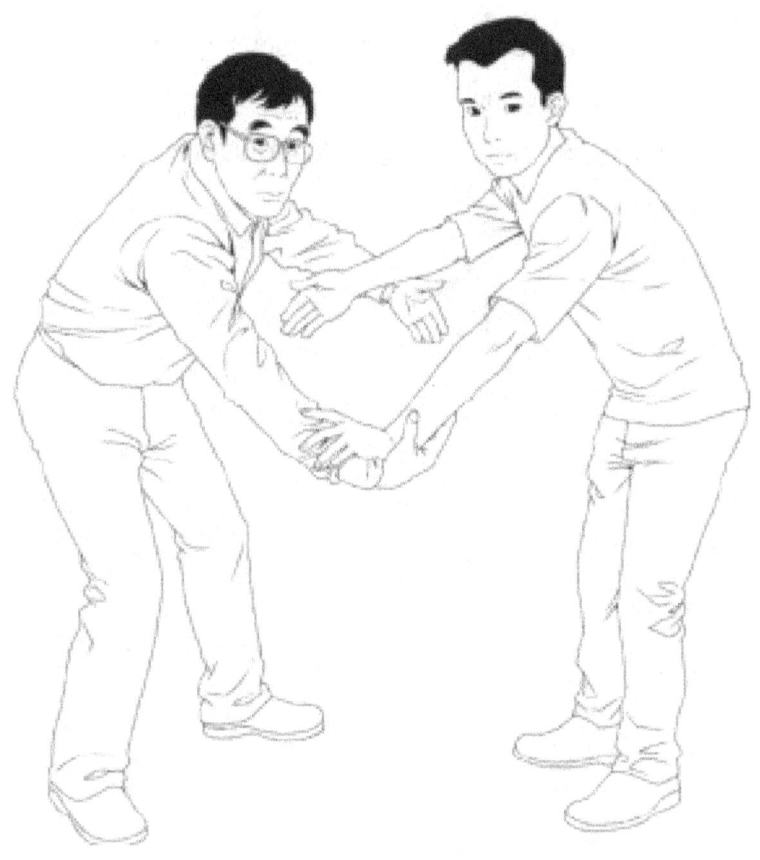

Carrying Method: Sedan Chair Carry

This method is suitable for conscious but physically weak victims.

Two rescuers face each other. Each rescuer grips their own left wrist with their right hand, and then both rescuers clasp each other's right wrist, forming a "hand seat" for the victim to sit on. The victim places their arms around the rescuers' necks for support. The rescuers then slowly stand up in unison, stepping first with their outer legs while maintaining synchronized movements to transport the victim safely.

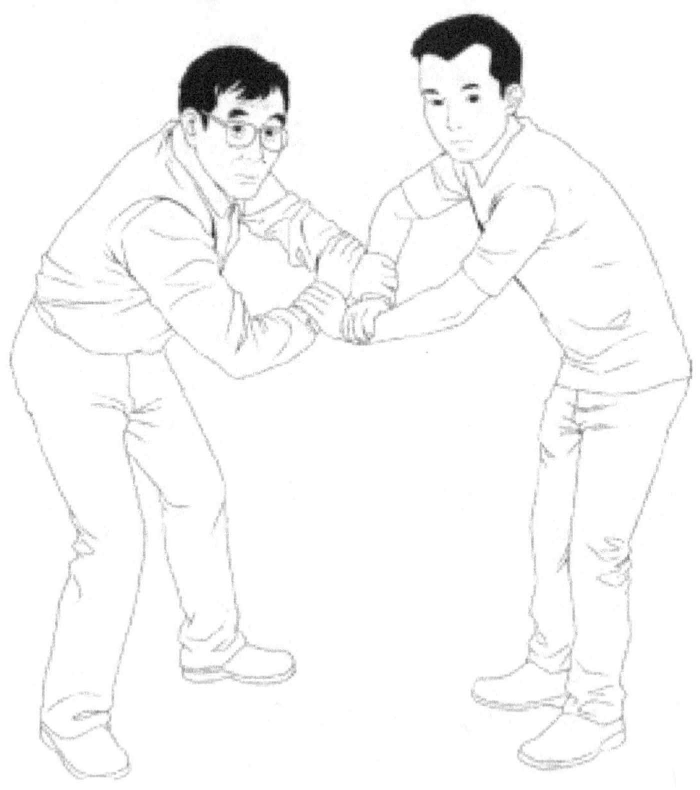

Two-Person Cart Carry Method
This method is suitable for unconscious victims, but must not be used for those with spinal or limb fractures.

Procedure:

- One rescuer stands behind the victim, threading both arms under the victim's armpits to support their chest, ensuring the victim's arms are crossed between their legs.
- The second rescuer faces forward with their back to the victim, positioning themselves between the victim's legs, then lifts the legs.
- Both rescuers, working in tandem—one at the front and one at the back—transport the victim.

Important Note:
Never move someone suspected of a spinal injury lightly. Here's an incident highlighting this:

During July or August one year, I received an emergency call and rushed to the scene. I found a young man lying on the ground—he had fallen from a building while installing an air conditioner due to improper operation. Although conscious, the man kept complaining of severe back pain. Upon inspection, I noticed abnormal protrusions along his spine, and he expressed pain when I pressed the area, unable to move—he had sustained a spinal injury.

Severe spinal injuries can damage the spinal

cord, leading to sensory and motor dysfunction, urinary and bowel incontinence, and sexual dysfunction. This makes emergency care at the scene critical. Professional care involves securing the neck with a cervical collar and using specialized equipment such as a spine board, scoop stretcher, or vacuum mattress. But in the absence of such equipment, the best approach is not to move the victim at all.

I firmly oppose untrained individuals from attempting to move a person with spinal injuries. Not moving them prevents further injury, while improper handling can worsen the condition or even threaten the victim's life.

Unlike cardiac arrest or major arterial bleeding, where immediate intervention is critical to prevent death, spinal injuries do not cause immediate fatality. Waiting for professional emergency responders is essential in such cases.

If you suspect a spinal injury from incidents like falls or traffic accidents, do not move the victim. Keep them still, prevent others from moving them, and call emergency services immediately.

Points to Remember During Emergency Transport:

1. Monitor the victim's condition closely, including consciousness, breathing, pulse, blood pressure, and the appearance of the injured area (e.g., color, temperature, bleeding).

2. For victims in shock, keep them in a supine position to ensure adequate blood flow to the brain.

3. Prevent airway obstruction in unconscious victims from vomit or secretions, and remove dentures if present.

4. For chest injuries, place the victim in a semi-sitting position.

5. For abdominal injuries:

   - If the wound is vertical: Keep the victim in a flat-lying position with legs straight.

   - If the wound is horizontal: Bend the legs to avoid wound expansion.

6. For victims with tourniquets, ensure proper tension and loosen the tourniquet every 40–50 minutes to prevent tissue damage.

7. Do not allow food or drink for victims needing surgery to prevent vomiting during anesthesia and the risk of aspiration pneumonia.

8. Provide appropriate warmth or cooling measures depending on the season.

How to Perform Self-Rescue and Mutual Aid During Major Catastrophic Accidents

In modern society, accidents such as traffic collisions, construction or mining incidents, terrorist attacks, and natural disasters occur frequently, placing everyone at risk.

According to the 2011 Injury Prevention Report released by the Ministry of Health, around 200 million people are injured annually in China, resulting in 700,000–750,000 deaths, accounting for 9% of the total population and making injuries the fifth leading cause of death after four major diseases. Fatal injuries—such as traffic accidents, suicides, drownings, poisonings, and falls—constitute approximately 70% of all injury-related deaths. Additionally, 62 million people require medical care annually, with direct medical expenses totaling 65 billion yuan, and economic losses from missed work exceeding 6 billion yuan.

Of all injury-related deaths:
- 50% occur within the first few minutes due to the victim's heart or breathing stopping abruptly, sometimes as fast as acute myocardial infarction or even faster than a stroke.
- 30% occur within 2–3 hours.
- 20% result from infections, organ failure, or complications weeks after the injury.

The three main causes of rapid death from seemingly minor injuries are asphyxiation, hemorrhagic shock, and severe damage to vital organs.

When a major disaster causes mass casualties, the following six steps should guide rescue efforts:

Six Key Steps for Rescue During a Catastrophe

1. Ensure Personal Safety

Before helping others, first observe the surrounding environment to ensure your own safety. If rescuers get injured, they may become a burden instead of providing assistance.

2. Protect Yourself

Take precautions to avoid becoming a victim. For example, wear a gas mask when entering a fire or gas-leak site. If you must come into contact with an injured person's blood, first ensure your hands have no open wounds, and ideally wear rubber gloves.

3. Identify Yourself

Introduce yourself to the injured person and inform them that you are there to help. This reassurance will gain their trust and make subsequent rescue efforts smoother.

4. Assess the Victim's Condition

Quickly evaluate the injury and, based on the circumstances, use a safe and efficient method to move the victim away from the danger zone.

5. Provide First Aid at a Safe Location

Once in a safe area, stop bleeding, protect wounds, or immobilize fractures to reduce the risk of shock and complications. These efforts are crucial in stabilizing the victim's condition and reducing mortality, buying time for professional rescuers to arrive.

6. Call Emergency Services (120)

Call for medical assistance immediately. If others are present, ask someone else to make the call while you continue assisting the victim. Use your phone's speaker mode if you are alone to free your hands.

Special Guidelines for Earthquakes and Fires

1. Earthquake Survival and Self-Rescue
In the aftermath of an earthquake, some survivors may be trapped under rubble, surrounded by darkness and fear. Before rescuers arrive, knowledge of first aid can be life-saving.

- Stay Calm: Clear your mind and try to free your limbs. Ensure your airway is open by loosening clothing around the neck and using fabric to cover your nose and mouth to prevent inhaling dust, as asphyxiation can cause death within minutes.

- Stabilize Debris: If you cannot escape immediately, try to secure any unstable debris to prevent further collapse. Avoid excessive movement to conserve energy and wait for rescuers.

- Signal for Help: Instead of shouting, which wastes energy, tap on nearby pipes or walls to alert rescuers to your location. Use moderate force to avoid triggering further collapse.

If bleeding occurs, apply pressure to the wound to stop the bleeding.

Remember, humans can survive without food for up to seven days, but lack of water becomes life-threatening after three days. Therefore, collect any water you can find among the debris.

If a limb is trapped under heavy objects for an extended period, do not simply remove the object immediately. This can cause crush syndrome, a condition where damaged muscle cells release toxins such as myoglobin and potassium into the bloodstream, leading to heart suppression, kidney failure, and sudden death.

To prevent this:

- Immobilize the affected limb with a splint.
- Do not move or elevate the injured limb, apply a tourniquet, or massage the area to avoid releasing toxins.
- Wait for professional rescue teams to manage the situation properly.

---

2. Fire Emergency Response
In a fire, avoid running or shouting, as it may cause inhalation burns. Such burns lead to rapid swelling of the airway, resulting in asphyxiation. Use a wet towel to cover your nose and mouth to prevent inhaling toxic gases.

How to Use a Wet Towel Properly:
Wrap the towel around your hand first, then use it to cover your nose and mouth. If you directly cover your face, your instinctive reaction to heat may cause you to pull the towel away, exposing your airway to burns or toxic gases. You can also dampen the towel after wrapping it around your hand for added protection.

If your clothes catch fire:

- Stop, drop, and roll to extinguish the flames.
- Use water, sand, or a fire extinguisher to put out the fire based on the situation.
- After escaping the fire, seek medical attention immediately.

By following these steps during disasters like earthquakes or fires, you can improve your chances of survival and help others effectively while waiting for professional assistance.

Chapter 5: Childhood Accidents – The Moment When Parents' First Aid Knowledge is Put to the Test

70% of childhood accidents happen at home.

Why dedicate a chapter to child first aid? It's not because the methods for child and adult first aid differ significantly, but rather due to the unique characteristics of children as a group.

Children develop rapidly. A newborn can't even turn its head, but soon enough, they can walk. According to infant development milestones, babies "can lift their heads by 2 months, roll over by 4 months, sit up by 6 months, roll around by 7 months, crawl by 8 months, and walk by 1 year old." At each stage, children may face different dangers.

Before 4 months, babies cannot roll over. At this stage, if a baby accidentally covers their mouth and nose with clothes, towels, or blankets, they cannot pull these items away or move, which could lead to suffocation. After 4 months, when babies can roll over, and by 8 months, when they start crawling, the risk of falling from the bed increases significantly. In reality, very few children have never fallen off the bed.

After the age of 1, children gain the ability to walk independently. With this expanded range of movement, the potential hazards they encounter also increase, leading to frequent incidents of burns, electric shocks, and other accidents.

Children aged 2 to 3 are highly curious, energetic, and lack good judgment, yet they are extremely confident and bold, often resulting in accidents.

By the time they reach elementary and middle school, as children's knowledge, experiences, independence, and range of activities grow, so does their exposure to danger, leading to more frequent accidents such as drowning and car accidents.

Furthermore, children often lack life experience and an awareness of danger. Their ability to discern and anticipate hazards is weaker than that of adults, and they are slower to react to dangerous situations. This lack of knowledge and skills in avoiding danger and escaping from peril is another major reason for childhood accidents. For example, when crossing the street, adults can judge whether an oncoming car poses a threat, whether they should hurry or stop to let the car pass. Children, however, are unable to do this, which is why they are much more likely to be hit by cars than adults.

A few years ago, I read a report that stated over 2.4 million children under the age of 14 in China die from accidental injuries each year. What does this mean? It means that hundreds of thousands of families suffer immense grief every year, with the sorrow potentially lasting for generations.

In my emergency medical career, I have rescued countless critically ill patients, but what pains me the most is witnessing children suffer accidental injuries or even die. For instance, two- or three-year-old children choking on peanuts, seeds, or jelly; children burned or scalded due to parental negligence; or children falling from buildings, drowning during summer play, and so on. These accidents can lead to irreversible tragedies.

Data shows that 70% of childhood accidents occur at home. Foreign body choking, burns, and drowning are leading causes of injury and death among children.

This raises an important question: Why, despite improving living conditions, are the factors threatening children's safety increasing? As guardians, why is parental protection so weak?

In my opinion, one reason is that many parents lack a sense of guardianship. Many of today's young parents, born in the 1980s and 1990s, are often only children themselves. Even as parents, they may struggle to take care of themselves, let alone their children, and their inexperience is exacerbated by being first-time parents. If grandparents take on caregiving duties, while they may have more experience, outdated caregiving practices and slower reactions can still inadvertently lead to harm.

More importantly, many parents don't know how to provide first aid when accidents happen, or they rely solely on experience and intuition, often missing the best window for treatment or even worsening the child's injuries. By the time regret sets in, it is often too late.

Emergency Scene Example

I recall one time when a mother had just filled a thermos with hot water and placed it on a chest of drawers, thinking that since her child was only 1 year old, they couldn't possibly reach it. But as soon as she walked a few steps away, she heard a loud "thud" followed by the child crying. What happened? The thermos had fallen, and the hot water had splashed all over the child. The thermos was placed high, so how did it fall? The answer was the tablecloth on the chest of drawers. The child had tugged on the tablecloth, causing the thermos to tumble down. Don't underestimate a tablecloth. I've also encountered cases where children pulled on tablecloths, causing knives or scissors to fall, leading to facial cuts or even head injuries.

When I asked the parents, they all said they

never imagined such a thing could happen. That's why I suggest that families with young children avoid using tablecloths altogether, just in case.

In addition to avoiding tablecloths, there are many other details to consider in creating a safe home environment. For example, is it necessary to install window guards? If you have children at home, regardless of what floor you live on, windows and balconies should be fitted with guards, not just for burglary prevention, but primarily for the child's safety. We often hear stories of children falling from several stories or even dozens of floors, with tragic consequences. Moreover, installing guards isn't just a matter of putting them up—it's crucial to pay attention to details. For example, guards should either be fully enclosed or at least 1.1 meters high, as anything lower could allow a child to climb over. The gap between bars should not exceed 11 cm, or the child might slip through. Additionally, the guards should be vertical rather than horizontal; otherwise, they might become a ladder for the child to climb.

For dedicated children's activity areas, such as kindergartens, I recommend using wooden floors with carpets, and all furniture should have rounded corners. A child falling on a cement floor is undoubtedly more serious than falling on a carpeted wooden floor. Rounded furniture corners are also much safer for children than sharp ones.

These are basic safety measures to protect children—who could say they're not important? Without them, children are at greater risk. As parents, we must stay extra vigilant. From the moment a child is born, many parents start thinking about nutrition and early education, but compared to these, the child's safety and health should always come first.

Instilling First Aid Awareness and Safety Knowledge in Children from an Early Age

An ancient saying goes: "Prepare well and you will succeed, fail to prepare and you will fail."

A correspondent for *Life Times* once wrote an article titled *First Aid Skills Everyone Must Learn Before 18*, which compared first aid education in China and the U.S., making me realize that the most significant gap in Chinese school education is first aid training.

In the U.S., the law mandates that every citizen must master all basic first aid skills before the age of 18. Parents abroad start educating their children about dangers between the ages of 2 and 6, teaching them that playing with knives can cause cuts, playing with fire can burn the skin, and putting plastic bags over their heads can suffocate them. Parents not only tell their children what is dangerous but also let them experience these dangers firsthand and explain how to avoid them. These lessons are crucial in helping children develop a sense of safety from an early age.

In elementary school, while children may not yet have learned first aid, teachers in other countries teach them how to call 911 (the U.S. emergency hotline). They are instructed to clearly state the patient's name, gender, and age. If they are home alone, after calling, they should unlock the front door, and if it's nighttime, turn on all the lights to help the ambulance find them quickly. They are also taught to describe the emergency situation as clearly as possible, such as whether the patient is unconscious or experiencing chest pain. Most importantly, they are instructed to specify the location where they are waiting for the ambulance, such as near a tall or landmark building. Teachers emphasize that children should know the name of their neighborhood or the street corner where they are located to assist the ambulance, as emergency vehicles can stop anywhere without being restricted by traffic rules. Children are encouraged to actively help guide the rescue team to the patient, which can save valuable time.

This kind of first aid education plays a significant role in fostering a sense of first aid awareness in children, something that can benefit them for life. As a result, the death rate due to first aid mistakes in the U.S. is much lower than in China.

As mentioned earlier, accidental injuries have become the leading cause of death among children. Parents cannot always be by their children's side to shield them from every risk. Therefore, parents should help their children develop a sense of danger from an early age and teach them correct first aid knowledge at the right time. As children grow, this not only helps them avoid risks but also enables them to acquire essential first aid awareness and skills, allowing them to help themselves and others in times of danger or physical distress.

Moreover, parents must understand that actions speak louder than words when it comes to cultivating safety awareness in children. Children are naturally curious and want to touch and explore everything, whether it's electrical outlets or gas stoves. Unfortunately, this curiosity leads to many accidents each year, such as burns or electrocution. Many of us have heard stories about children setting their homes on fire with matches, and I have even heard of cases where children urinated on electrical appliances and were electrocuted to death.

While it is essential to nurture children's curiosity, it is equally important to protect them from danger.

For example, during home renovations, electrical outlets should be installed at least 1.6 meters above the ground to prevent children from reaching them, and wiring should not be exposed. Electric fans, heaters, and other appliances should be equipped with protective covers. Matches, lighters, and other dangerous items should be kept out of children's sight and reach. Children should also be kept away from gas stoves and gas water heaters. As children grow older, parents should educate them about fire and electrical safety and teach them the proper use of household appliances.

Generally, visual examples leave a more profound impression on children. For instance, taking children to see burn patients in a hospital might be more effective than telling them a thousand times not to touch boiling water.

"Impulsiveness is the Devil": Using the Right Approach to Educate Children

In addition to cultivating first aid awareness in children from a young age, many parents need to develop their own first aid awareness—not just knowledge of first aid techniques, but also basic medical knowledge. Some parents are what I call "medically ignorant." The most heartbreaking cases I've encountered are when parents, in disciplining their children, are too heavy-handed, pushing them to the brink, and when something goes wrong, their ignorance leads to tragic consequences.

Emergency Scene

I once encountered such a case. It was around 3 a.m. when I arrived at the patient's home. Upon entering, I saw a boy, about 8 years old, lying on the bed, without a heartbeat or breathing, his body already cold. His father sat nearby in shock, pulling at his hair, muttering, "How could this happen? How could this happen?" In this situation, I didn't have time to comfort the parent. I immediately started resuscitating the child while asking questions.

"What happened?"
"I killed him."
"What do you mean you killed him? Was it something to do with work or some incident?"
"I hit him, beat him to death."
"Where did you hit him?"
"Just his buttocks, nowhere else."
"When did you hit him?"
"Around 7 p.m. last night."

It had already been more than eight hours. This was a single-parent family. The father, frustrated by his child's disobedience, had taken a wooden board and harshly punished him. After the beating, he sent the child to bed, but by the time he checked on him in the middle of the night, it was too late.

I quickly removed the boy's pants and saw that his buttocks were severely bruised and swollen, with large areas of subcutaneous bleeding on both sides. The blows had been too harsh.

Even though we knew the boy couldn't be revived, we still made every effort to save him, but in the end, he didn't make it. The father, filled with regret, repeatedly banged his head against the wall, the sound echoing in the room: "I never thought beating his buttocks could kill him. I just wanted to teach this ungrateful child a lesson. If I had known this would happen, I would never have hit him." But there's no medicine for regret, and this incident illustrates one key lesson: Don't hit children—not even on the buttocks.

Many people believe that hitting the buttocks is harmless because it's "well-padded." However, it is precisely because the buttocks have thick muscles that serious injuries can occur. Severe blows can cause muscle cells to rupture, releasing large amounts of potassium ions and myoglobin. The potassium ions can lead to cardiac arrest, and when myoglobin enters the bloodstream and passes through the kidneys, it can block the renal tubules, causing acute kidney failure. This is similar to what happens to earthquake victims who die after being trapped under debris for a long time, even after being rescued.

In situations like this, if parents had basic medical knowledge and noticed something was wrong with the child, they could have stopped in time and taken the child to the hospital for examination. The doctors might have been able to intervene and save the child. Of course, if parents didn't resort to physical punishment in the first place, such tragedies wouldn't happen.

Emergency Scene

I recall another case where a 12-year-old boy argued with his father. As the argument escalated, the father, overwhelmed with anger, grabbed a teapot and threw it at his son. The teapot struck the boy's forehead, eyebrow, and eyelid, leaving a gaping 5-centimeter cut that bled profusely, soaking his clothes in blood. The teapot shattered on the floor. When I arrived, the boy's mother was pressing her hand against his wound, but blood was still flowing through her fingers.

The mother was scolding the father, who sat silently smoking, saying nothing.

I quickly applied sterile dressing to stop the bleeding, and after a few minutes, the bleeding ceased. I then bandaged the wound.

I quietly told the father, "That was close. If it had been just a little lower, his eye could have been blinded." I could see the regret, guilt, and pain in the father's eyes.

Another case that left a deep impression on me occurred one Monday morning. We arrived at a home to find a 13-year-old boy lying in bed, barely responsive. I called out to him loudly, and though he could open his eyes, his expression was dull, his hands trembled, and he answered questions slowly. He said he was sweating, dizzy, lightheaded, weak, and had numbness in his limbs.

After questioning, we found out that the boy had failed two subjects on an exam, and as punishment, his parents had not allowed him to eat for more than two days. I quickly tested his blood sugar, which was 2.6 mmol/L (normal fasting blood glucose is 3.8–6.1 mmol/L), indicating severe hypoglycemia due to hunger. I immediately administered a 60 ml intravenous injection of 50% glucose. The boy quickly regained some strength, and we took him to the hospital for further treatment.

Ultimately, when it comes to educating children, parents need to reason with them and use civilized methods, avoiding violence. Whether hitting the head or the buttocks, both can cause problems, and once something goes wrong, it's often irreversible, leaving parents with nothing but regret.

Foreign Objects in the Airway: The Heimlich Maneuver Can Solve It All

Festive occasions, such as holidays, are also the busiest times for emergency centers. Families gather together, and those who usually don't drink may have a few drinks out of joy. Children receive everyone's attention—grandma holds them, grandpa kisses them, and uncles play with them, bringing laughter to all. But often, it's at such moments that hidden dangers arise!

During the 2014 Spring Festival, a piece of news went viral on Weibo: A 2.5-year-old child was fed a pistachio by a relative, and the nut accidentally entered the child's trachea. The child immediately had difficulty breathing, and their face turned blue. The family, terrified, rushed the child to the hospital. Despite undergoing an emergency tracheotomy, the child could not be saved.

Many blamed the relative for being careless, but

if we think carefully, how many people truly knew beforehand not to randomly feed children? How many people were familiar with the Heimlich maneuver? If just one person in that family had known how to perform the Heimlich maneuver and applied it in time, perhaps the pistachio wouldn't have claimed the child's life.

Studies show that accidents are the leading cause of death for children aged 0–14, with airway obstruction from foreign objects being a major cause of choking-related deaths. Children between 0 and 4 years old are particularly at risk.

Many may ask, why is it so easy for foreign objects to enter a child's airway? And why is the situation so critical once it happens? The answer lies in the unique "geography" of the throat.

The throat is where the airway and esophagus run parallel. The airway (trachea) is responsible for inhaling and exhaling air, and should only allow air to pass—no liquids or solids. The esophagus, on the other hand, is the passage for food, and air should not enter it. If too much air enters the esophagus, it can lead to abdominal pain or bloating.

The "epiglottis," a flap at the entrance of the larynx, separates air and food. When it is open, we can breathe; when it closes, water and food are prevented from entering the airway. Generally, the epiglottis functions automatically, controlled by the nervous system. However, since children's nervous systems are not fully developed, their swallowing reflexes are not yet mature, making them prone to "taking the wrong route"—allowing liquids or solids to enter the airway.

Once a foreign object enters the airway, two outcomes are possible: complete airway obstruction or partial obstruction. Partial obstruction is more common and is something most people have experienced—such as when drinking water and accidentally choking. Typically, we start coughing violently, which is a protective reflex. The coughing uses air from the lungs to expel the foreign object, clearing the obstruction and saving us from danger. In cases of choking on blood or vomit, placing the person in a head-down, feet-up position can help drain the liquid from the airway using gravity.

If a foreign object enters the airway, children will display certain symptoms that parents need to recognize immediately to provide timely first aid. If the object is large and causes a complete obstruction, meaning the airway is entirely blocked, the body cannot exchange gases with the outside environment. The child will exhibit the "three no's" symptoms: unable to cough, unable to breathe, and unable to speak. Soon after, they will struggle to breathe, their face will turn blue, they'll become restless, and severe oxygen deprivation to the brain will follow. Consciousness will be lost, and the heart will soon stop. The situation is extremely critical.

If the foreign object is smaller, the child will begin coughing violently and experience difficulty breathing. The object may be expelled through coughing or may remain lodged, potentially worsening the blockage, which could eventually cause the child to stop breathing and lead to cardiac arrest.

If the foreign object enters one side of the airway

(most commonly the right), the child may develop symptoms like coughing and wheezing, which could later lead to lung infections. If the foreign object contains fatty acids, such as peanuts or almonds, the airway inflammation will be more severe, causing coughing and phlegm. If small objects like buttons or marbles are inhaled, there may be no symptoms at first, but after weeks or months, the child may experience recurrent fever, coughing, and phlegm, potentially leading to chronic bronchitis, pneumonia, or bronchiectasis. If a child suffers from recurrent bronchitis or pneumonia, parents should take them to the hospital as soon as possible.

In my opinion, airway obstruction due to foreign objects is one of the most dangerous emergencies, second only to cardiac arrest. It requires immediate action to save lives. So how do we perform first aid? The internationally recognized method for removing foreign objects from the airway is the Heimlich maneuver.

Dr. Henry Heimlich, an American surgeon, was shocked to discover that airway obstruction was the sixth leading cause of accidental death in the U.S. in the late 1960s. At the time, doctors commonly used back blows or tried to manually remove the object from the throat, often pushing it deeper with little success.

After years of research, Heimlich developed the "abdominal thrust" technique. In October 1975, the American Medical Association named the method after him and widely promoted it through newspapers and television. By 1979, just four years later, over 3,000 people had been saved by this method in the U.S. alone. To date, the Heimlich maneuver has saved at least 100,000 lives worldwide, and *The Guinness Book of World Records* hails Dr. Heimlich as the person who has saved the most lives.

Heimlich Maneuver for Adult Airway Obstruction

The abdominal thrust method works by forcefully elevating the diaphragm, causing a sudden increase in lung pressure. This generates an artificial cough, using airflow from the lungs to expel the foreign object from the airway, thereby clearing the obstruction. There are two variations: the standing or seated abdominal thrust for conscious adults, and the lying-down abdominal thrust for unconscious adults.

The standing or seated abdominal thrust is suitable for conscious adult patients. The patient stands, and the rescuer stands behind them, placing one leg forward between the patient's legs and the other leg back for stability. The rescuer wraps their arms around the patient's waist, makes a fist with one hand, and positions it just above the navel. The other hand covers the fist. The rescuer then quickly and forcefully thrusts upward and inward toward the patient's abdomen, repeating the maneuver until the foreign object is expelled or the patient loses consciousness.

The lying-down abdominal thrust is for unconscious patients. The rescuer straddles the patient's thighs, places the heel of one hand on the center of the abdomen just above the navel, overlaps the other hand on top, and delivers rapid, forceful upward thrusts. After every five thrusts, the rescuer checks the patient's mouth for any expelled objects. If the object is visible, it should be removed immediately. If not, the process is repeated until the obstruction is cleared.

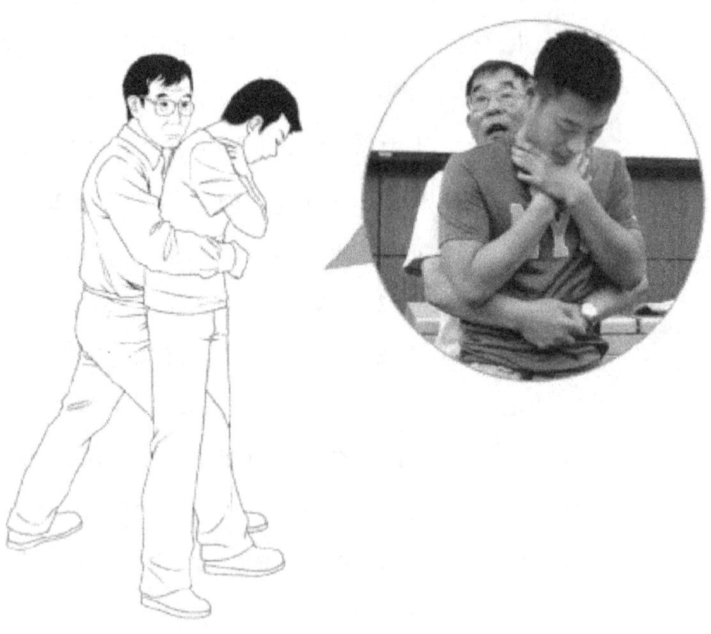

Chest Thrust Method: For Obese Individuals or Pregnant Women

This method is suitable for obese individuals or pregnant women, with two variations: the standing or seated chest thrust and the lying-down chest thrust.

Standing or Seated Chest Thrust

This is used for conscious obese individuals or pregnant women. The patient should be standing or seated, while the rescuer stands behind the patient, placing one leg between the patient's legs in a lunge position, with the other leg extended back for stability. The rescuer then wraps their arms around the patient's chest, making a fist with one hand and placing it between the patient's breasts (at the center of the chest between the nipples). The other hand stabilizes the fist. The rescuer then delivers quick, forceful thrusts backward toward the chest until the foreign object is expelled from the airway or the patient loses consciousness.

Why position the leg between the patient's legs? First, it helps maintain stability. Second, if the patient loses consciousness, they can sit on the rescuer's leg, allowing the rescuer to gently lower them to the ground and continue the rescue without causing injury from a fall. This method is both energy-efficient and safe for the patient.

Lying-Down Chest Thrust

This variation is for unconscious obese individuals or pregnant women. The rescuer kneels beside the patient and places the heel of one hand on the center of the chest (midway between the nipples). The other hand is placed on top, fingers interlocked. With arms mostly straight, the rescuer delivers strong, vertical downward thrusts. After every five thrusts, the rescuer checks the patient's mouth for expelled foreign objects. If an object is found, it should be removed immediately; if not, the process is repeated until the airway is cleared.

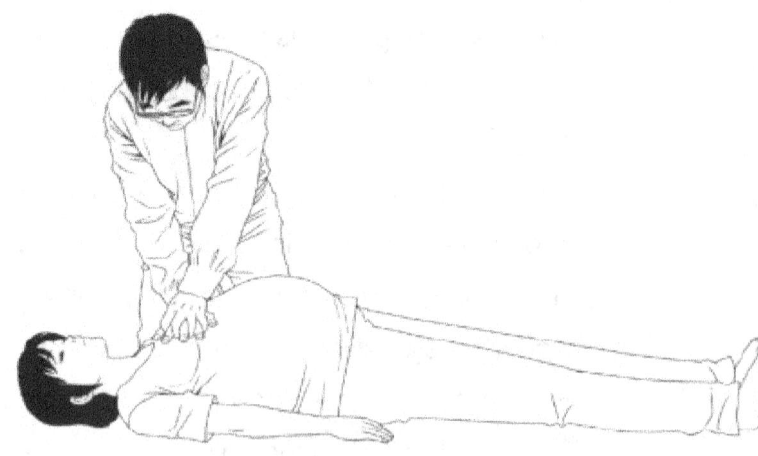

Self-Rescue for Adult Airway Obstruction

If a foreign object obstructs your airway and no one is around to help, it is crucial to act quickly within two to three minutes while you are still conscious. You can perform self-rescue by using a sturdy surface, such as the edge of a table, chair, bed frame, or a wide windowsill. Position the edge at the area two fingers above your navel, tilt your head back to straighten your airway, and extend your neck. Then, forcefully thrust your abdomen against the surface to create pressure and attempt to expel the object from your airway.

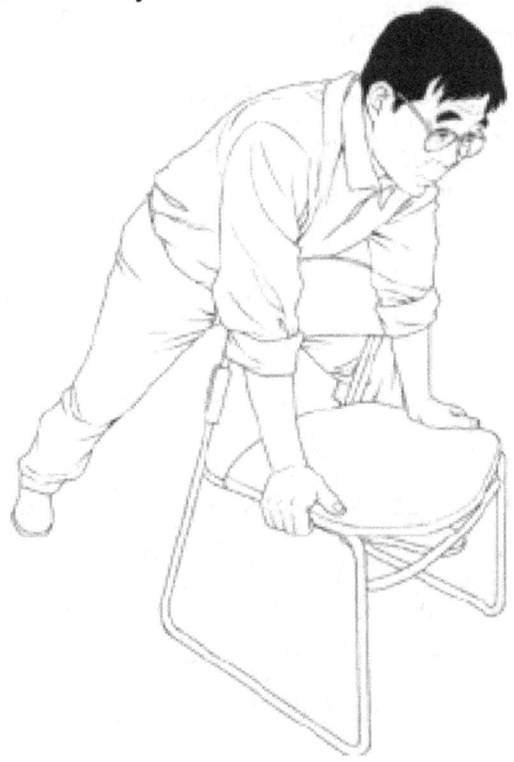

Airway Obstruction Management for Infants

When an infant experiences airway obstruction due to a foreign object, two methods can be used: back blows and chest thrusts. With one hand, secure the infant's head and neck, positioning the infant face down with their head lower than their hips. Using the heel of your other hand, deliver five firm back blows to the area between the infant's shoulder blades. Then, turn the infant face up, again keeping the head lower than the hips. Use your index and middle fingers to apply five quick thrusts to the lower half of the infant's breastbone. These two methods should be alternated repeatedly until the object is expelled.

The following steps outline the process in more detail:

1. Back Blow Method

The rescuer should kneel on one leg or sit down, placing the infant's abdomen across their thigh, with the infant's head lower than the hips. One hand should support the infant's head and neck, keeping the face down. Using the heel of the other hand, deliver five strong blows between the shoulder blades. After each round of blows, check to see if the object has been expelled. If not, continue repeating the process.

This method works by utilizing both the force of gravity and the vibrations caused by the blows.

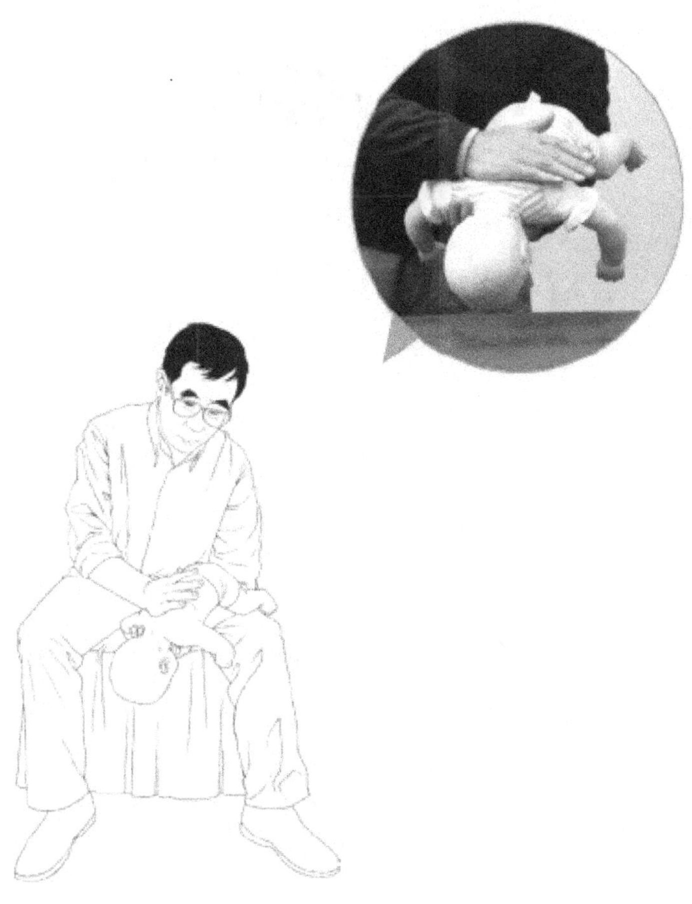

2. Chest Thrust Method

Support the infant securely and turn them face up. Using your index and middle fingers, apply five quick thrusts to the lower half of the infant's breastbone (sternum). This method can be alternated with the back blow method until the foreign object is expelled.

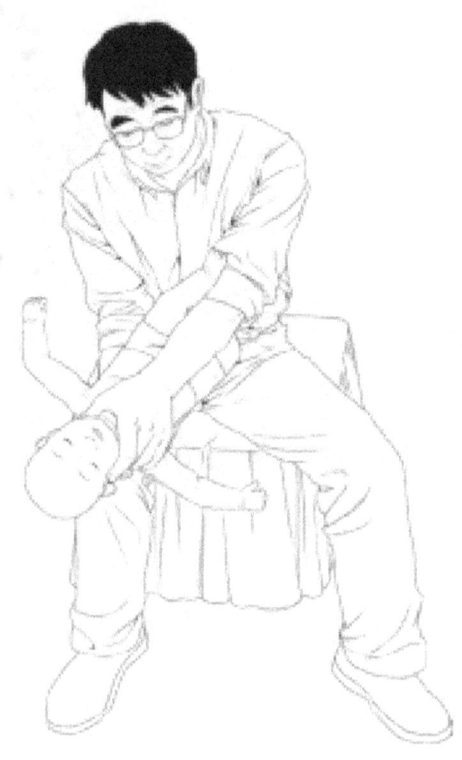

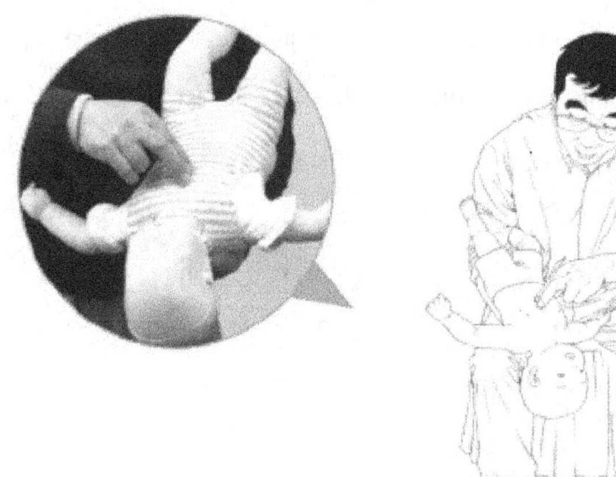

3. Abdominal Thrust Method

For infants, the rescuer positions themselves behind the infant, either sitting in a chair, standing and squatting, or kneeling on one knee. Place two or three fingers of one hand horizontally just above the infant's navel, and then place two or three fingers of the other hand on top of the first hand. Deliver repeated upward and inward thrusts towards the infant's diaphragm.

The lying-down abdominal thrust method can also be used for infants (similar to the adult version). If the infant loses consciousness, immediately lay the infant flat on the ground. Straddle the infant's body, place the heel of one hand just above the navel, and perform five to six forceful thrusts. After each set, check the infant's mouth for any foreign objects. If none are visible, continue repeating the thrusts until the obstruction is cleared.

Jelly "Choking": Using the Negative Pressure Suction Method

According to statistics from Taiwan, 91.2% of airway obstructions are caused by food, with the most common culprits being peanuts, sunflower seeds, cherimoya seeds, beans, candy, and fruit pits. Additionally, some toys like marbles and pins can also lead to choking. Over the years, we've encountered many cases of airway obstructions in children caused by various objects, including button batteries, keys, nails, and different fruit pits and nuts. While apple or pear pits usually don't cause fatalities, a lychee or apricot pit in the airway can be deadly. Also, when parents force-feed medication to a crying and uncooperative child by pinching their nose, the medicine can enter the airway, which is extremely dangerous. Parents must be cautious. Additionally, children should not drink or eat while laughing or crying, as this can cause food to enter the airway and lead to choking.

Some children also enjoy putting small objects up their noses, like peanuts or toy parts. If the object remains in the nasal cavity, parents can hold the child's head slightly down and gently tap their back to encourage the object to come out. If this doesn't work, a doctor should be consulted immediately. The danger arises when the object moves deeper into the nasal passage and enters the airway, which can be life-threatening.

Among all the potential airway obstructions, jelly is the most dangerous. Each year, many children die from choking on jelly. The government has introduced regulations stating that cup-shaped jelly products must have an inner cup diameter of at least 3.5 cm, and the content of long or strip-shaped jelly must be at least 6 cm in length. However, smaller jellies are still sold in the market, which poses a hidden danger. In a moment of inattention, children can ingest these "deadly jellies."

Emergency Scene

I once encountered such a situation. The parents were busy running their restaurant and often let their child play by themselves. One day, a customer noticed that the child playing nearby had turned pale and was waving their arms frantically. Seeing an empty jelly cup on the table, someone shouted, "The child is choking on jelly!" Within two minutes, the child began to exhibit symptoms of choking—rapid breathing, a bluish-purple face, and visible distress. The father was on the verge of tears, panicking over what to do.

The tiny jelly posed a problem for everyone at the scene. The child's condition worsened, with their lips turning dark purple and their eyes staring blankly. Someone attempted back blows, but the jelly did not come out. The parents rushed the child to the hospital, but tragically, by the time they arrived, the child had stopped breathing—dead from jelly-induced suffocation.

There have been far too many such incidents. Jelly, in particular, is difficult to remove from the airway, even in a hospital setting. Jelly is soft and large, and tools like laryngoscopes, bronchoscopes, or tracheoscopes cannot easily remove it because it cannot be hooked or clamped.

Jelly has another dangerous characteristic: it is soft and can change shape. If a button enters the trachea, it retains its size and shape and may not completely block the airway. The child may survive for some time. But jelly can mold to the shape of the airway and completely block it, leading to rapid suffocation.

If jelly enters a child's airway, in addition to using the Heimlich maneuver, I have a special technique to teach you: the Negative Pressure Suction Method. It is crucial for parents to learn this method. I once shared it on Sina Weibo, and two parents later told me that they used it to save their children's lives.

Specific Steps for the Negative Pressure Suction Method

1. Tilt the child's head back to straighten the

airway; otherwise, the jelly won't come out.

2. Seal the child's mouth with your mouth, pinch the child's nose shut, and suck forcefully to create negative pressure in the child's mouth. This suction can help pull the jelly out of the airway.

3. Once the jelly is in the mouth, turn the child's head to one side and use your fingers to carefully remove the jelly. Be careful not to push it deeper into the throat.

4. If the child is not breathing after removing the jelly, begin mouth-to-mouth resuscitation immediately, just like the technique used in CPR.

Additional Advice for Parents

Jelly has little nutritional value, and it's best not to give it to children. If they must have it, choose larger jellies to prevent them from swallowing it whole, or opt for jelly that can be sucked through a straw to reduce the risk. You can also break the jelly into smaller pieces with a spoon before giving it to children. This way, even if it enters the airway, the likelihood of a complete obstruction is lower. Also, never leave young children alone while eating jelly—always supervise them closely.

Drowning Rescue: Open the Airway, Perform Rescue Breathing, and Chest Compressions

Every summer, emergency centers see a spike in children brought in for drowning. Despite schools' safety warnings before the holidays, some children still sneak off to swim in natural bodies of water like rivers and lakes. For example, nearly every year, children drown in Beijing's Shichahai Lake, and other natural waters present similar dangers.

In today's world, where most families only have one child, parents work hard to raise their children. A swimming accident would be a devastating loss. Parents must teach their children to have safety awareness, and if children want to swim, parents should take them to regulated swimming pools and supervise them carefully.

Why do people drown?

Of course, not knowing how to swim is one reason, but there is a saying: "Those who drown are often good swimmers." So why do experienced swimmers drown?

1. Fatigue: Children often forget everything when playing, and before they realize it, they've been swimming for a long time and become tired. Excessive carbon dioxide exhalation can lead to respiratory alkalosis, causing dizziness and even convulsions. In severe cases, this can lead to loss of consciousness and drowning.

2. Cramps: Most people are familiar with this. Cold water can cause leg cramps while swimming, making it difficult to swim properly. Panic and fear can exacerbate the situation, leading to drowning.

3. Hunger: This is common among children. Many are so focused on playing that they skip meals before swimming, which can lead to low blood sugar, dizziness, and even loss of consciousness, resulting in drowning.

4. Illness: While less common in children, sudden illness can also lead to drowning, such as seizures or asthma attacks. Parents should be particularly cautious if their child has a medical condition like epilepsy or asthma.

Additionally, drinking alcohol before swimming is a common cause of drowning among teenagers, although it is rare in younger children.

From the moment a child starts drowning to the point of death, it only takes a few minutes. During this time, the child experiences intense fear and pain. Initially, the child will struggle to stay afloat, instinctively trying to breathe. Each time they surface, they manage to take a few breaths before sinking again. After several attempts, the child becomes exhausted and can no longer come up. The lack of oxygen, combined with the physical struggle and psychological panic, leads to severe brain hypoxia, loss of consciousness, and, eventually, the cessation of both breathing and heart function. Without immediate rescue, the child will soon die.

Why follow the ABC order?

For most cardiac arrests, the heart stops first, followed by breathing cessation, which is why we prioritize chest compressions first. However, in cases of drowning or respiratory-related cardiac arrest, such as asthma, the person stops breathing first, and the heart stops later. The cardiac arrest is a result of respiratory failure, so the key to resuscitation is to restore breathing. Of course, don't forget to call for emergency services while performing CPR. As we know, brain damage occurs if breathing and heart function stop for more than 4–6 minutes, and brain death occurs after 10 minutes. But for drowning victims, there's a reason not to give up easily, even if resuscitation seems delayed:

1. Diving Reflex: The diving reflex slows down the heart rate without immediately stopping it, ensuring that blood supply to the brain is maintained longer. Additionally, the reflex constricts blood vessels in less vital areas, redirecting blood flow to the brain and other vital organs. This extends the time during which the

brain can survive without oxygen.

2. Cold Water: Cold water can lower the body's metabolic rate and oxygen consumption, allowing the brain to tolerate a lack of oxygen for a longer period.

New Lifesaving Skills

How to Rescue a Drowning Child:

1. If the rescuer is a good swimmer, they should swim behind the child, hold the child's head to keep the nose and mouth above water, and use a backstroke technique to drag the child to shore. Alternatively, the rescuer can wrap their arms under the child's armpits, ensuring the child's head stays above water while dragging them to safety.

2. If the rescuer is not a strong swimmer, they should look for a long rope, stick, or bamboo pole, hold one end, and throw the other to the child, pulling them to safety. If no such objects are available, call for help immediately and avoid acting recklessly.

3. Once the child is pulled from the water, immediately begin CPR, following the ABC sequence: A = Airway, B = Breathing, C = Circulation. This means opening the airway first, followed by rescue breathing, and then chest compressions. This is different from the typical CAB sequence used in cardiac arrest situations, where compressions come first. For drowning victims, restoring breathing takes priority to increase the chances of survival.

Beware of Hidden Head and Neck Injuries in Drowning Children

When a child is rescued from drowning and initial first aid has been performed—restoring breathing and heartbeat—it may seem like the crisis is over. However, parents must remain vigilant for any potential injuries, especially to the head and neck. Sometimes, children who are playing recklessly dive headfirst into water, hitting their heads and causing the drowning. Scrapes, bruises, or even fractures are less of a concern than internal head injuries or cervical spine damage.

Additionally, there is a common belief that after rescuing a drowning person, you need to "drain water" from their body. This idea is often reinforced by news reports of people running around with a rescued child on their back to revive them. Let me clarify that such a child could likely have been saved without all the running; their breathing and heartbeat probably hadn't stopped, and they had only lost consciousness temporarily.

Should you drain water after rescuing a drowning child?

No! Why do many people think it's necessary? The academic understanding of this issue has evolved over time. Initially, it was believed that water needed to be drained from drowning victims. Later, it was thought that this applied only to saltwater drowning, not freshwater drowning. Now, it is agreed across the board that water drainage is not necessary at all. Here's why:

1. Some children don't actually inhale any water. At the moment they choke on water, the cold shock and panic cause the glottis to close, preventing water from entering the airway. In this case, there's no water in the lungs, so there's nothing to drain. However, because the glottis is closed, the child cannot exchange gases, leading to suffocation.

2. Even if water enters the airway, it can be

absorbed into the bloodstream without needing to be drained.

3. Draining water could cause secretions to enter the airway, which could actually induce choking and make the situation worse.

4. Draining water wastes time that could be used to perform CPR, which could be life-saving.

After rescuing a drowning child, instead of worrying about draining water, quickly assess the situation and follow the ABC sequence of CPR: open the Airway, perform Breathing, and then initiate Chest compressions to help the child recover as soon as possible.

A Specific Case: Bathtub Drowning

Parents also need to be cautious about drowning incidents in bathtubs. I once encountered a case where a family had a large, luxurious bathroom with an enamel bathtub about 60 cm high. One day, after filling the tub with water, the adults left the bathroom for a short while, and their child wandered in. By the time the parents realized, the child had drowned in the tub. Despite our efforts, we couldn't save the child. I suspect the child climbed one leg into the tub, slipped while trying to lift the other leg, and fell into the water. Being small and panicking, the child couldn't grab the edge of the tub to stand up, and drowned within moments.

Even if you don't have a bathtub at home, many people have washbasins for bathing children. If a basin is filled with water and a child falls in, submersion of the nose and mouth can cause suffocation, regardless of water depth. Water buckets can also pose a threat to small children—if they fall headfirst into a bucket, they can drown just as easily. Therefore, parents must always remain vigilant, never leaving water-filled containers unattended with children nearby.

Important Safety Tips

When preparing bathwater for a child, always fill the basin with cold water first, then add hot water. This is critical. We've encountered cases where a parent filled the basin with boiling water first and walked away to get cold water. Seeing the water, the child sat down in it and suffered severe burns, unable to sit for the rest of the summer due to the pain.

Monitoring a Rescued Drowning Child's Condition

Children who have suffered any type of injury, especially those who have been rescued from drowning, should be monitored closely for 24 hours. Parents need to observe the child's behavior and condition. If any of the following symptoms occur, they should take the child to the hospital immediately:

1. Crying inconsolably for more than 30 minutes.
2. Vomiting repeatedly (two or more times).
3. Blood or fluid draining from the nose or ears.
4. Bruising around the eyes.
5. Symptoms such as dizziness, nausea, vomiting, headaches, drowsiness, seizures, confusion, or decreased ability to speak or walk.

If the child is sleeping, parents should wake them every two hours. If the child cannot be awakened, they should be rushed to the hospital for evaluation.

Acute Carbon Monoxide Poisoning: Prevent Vomit-Induced Asphyxiation

Years ago, during the winter, many homes used coal stoves for heating, and we frequently rescued patients suffering from carbon monoxide poisoning. I recall one tragic case where over 10 people died. Nowadays, with central heating in most homes, fewer families use coal stoves, and cases of carbon monoxide poisoning have significantly decreased. However, improper installation or use of gas water heaters can still lead to carbon monoxide poisoning. In one incident, a mother and her child died because the mother used a gas water heater to bathe the child in a closed room without proper ventilation.

For those still using coal stoves, it's crucial to ensure that the chimney or vent is not blocked. But what should you do if you suspect someone has been poisoned by carbon monoxide?

There are some common folk remedies for carbon monoxide poisoning, but most are harmful and should not be used. Techniques like forcing the patient to drink vinegar or pickled cabbage soup not only fail to alleviate the poisoning but also increase the risk of asphyxiation.

Another folk remedy involves exposing the patient to the cold to "wake them up," but this is dangerous. As I mentioned earlier, keeping the patient warm is essential. After carbon monoxide poisoning, the body is already weak and vulnerable. Exposing the patient to the cold, especially in winter, can easily lead to pneumonia.

First Aid for Carbon Monoxide Poisoning

1. Lower your body position when entering the scene to avoid inhaling more carbon monoxide. Since carbon monoxide is lighter than air, it tends to be at the height of the breathing zone, so standing upright increases the risk of inhaling more of the toxic gas.

2. Ventilate the area immediately by opening windows to allow airflow, and move the patient outdoors. If the patient has mild poisoning, they often recover quickly after breathing fresh air. In winter, be sure to keep the patient warm to avoid further complications.

3. For an unconscious patient, ensure their airway is clear and prevent asphyxiation from vomit by placing them in a stable side-lying position. Immediately call emergency services (120) and transport the patient to the hospital for hyperbaric oxygen therapy.

Ingesting Household Items: When to Induce Vomiting

Accidental ingestion of medications, toxins, or household cleaning products is common, especially among children. Medications, in particular, pose a risk because many pills are coated with a sweet-tasting shell. Children may lick the pill and, finding it sweet, assume it's candy and consume it. In some cases, children have mistaken pesticides stored in soda bottles for drinks and taken a sip. There are also rare instances where children have ingested industrial sodium nitrite, mistaking it for table salt.

If you find that a child has ingested medication or poison, the first thing to check is whether the child is conscious. If the child is alert and responsive, induce vomiting immediately. Here's how:

- Induce vomiting by having the child drink about 300 ml of water (adjust the amount based on the child's size), and then use a non-sharp object, such as the handle of a toothbrush, to stimulate the child's gag reflex at the back of their throat, prompting them to vomit. Repeat the process a few times. This procedure, called "oral gastric lavage," mimics the process of stomach pumping in a hospital.

- Use lukewarm water, close to body temperature. If the water is too hot, it can dilate the capillaries in the stomach lining, promoting the absorption of toxins. If too cold, the stomach will contract, raising internal pressure and pushing the toxins into the intestines, making it harder to cleanse the stomach.

After inducing vomiting, take the child to the hospital immediately.

If the child is unconscious, do not attempt to induce vomiting, as this could lead to aspiration and asphyxiation. Instead, call emergency services and get the child to the hospital as quickly as possible.

How Poisonings Are Treated in the Hospital

In cases of poisoning, the best treatment is to use an antidote if one is available, such as methylene blue for sodium nitrite poisoning or pralidoxime for organophosphate poisoning. However, antidotes are available only for a limited number of toxins. Most cases of poisoning are treated symptomatically, with gastric lavage (stomach pumping) being a crucial step in treatment.

- If the child is brought to the hospital within six hours of ingestion, gastric lavage should be performed to remove as much of the toxin as possible before it's absorbed. After six hours, most toxins have already been absorbed, and stomach pumping becomes less effective.

- During gastric lavage, if the child is conscious, it's important to change their position frequently—from left to right side, and then to prone position—to ensure that all areas of the stomach are cleansed.

In some cases, poisoning can occur through skin

absorption, especially with substances like pesticides. If a child comes into contact with pesticides, remove their clothing immediately and wash their skin with warm water to reduce absorption.

Preventing Poisonings at Home

To avoid accidental ingestion, parents must ensure that medications, cleaning products, and other dangerous substances are stored out of children's reach. Never store these items in containers typically used for food or beverages. Every year, there are numerous heartbreaking cases where children mistakenly drink dangerous chemicals stored in beverage bottles.

If a child ingests weak alkaline or neutral detergents, these are usually not highly toxic. If the child consumes a small amount, induce vomiting and monitor for symptoms. If the ingestion was significant or the child displays serious symptoms, take them to the hospital for evaluation. Increasing fluid intake helps flush out the toxin.

If a child consumes corrosive substances like iodine, creosote, or strong acids, immediately have them drink a starch-rich solution, such as rice water or a slurry made of flour, to reduce damage to the stomach lining. If the substance ingested is strongly alkaline (e.g., toilet cleaner), give the child vinegar, lemon juice, or orange juice to neutralize the base. Conversely, if the child has ingested strong acids, like concentrated hydrochloric acid, give them baking soda or soapy water to neutralize the acid.

Important: If the child has ingested strong acids or bases, do not induce vomiting, as this can cause further damage to the digestive tract. After basic home treatment, take the child to the hospital immediately.

Key Points for Inducing Vomiting in Children

1. The amount of water given should be based on the child's weight. For adults, it's typically 300

ml; for smaller children, give an amount similar to what they would normally drink in a feeding.

2. Ensure that the child vomits the same amount they drank.

3. Save the vomit for the hospital, ideally in a glass container, as it can help doctors identify the toxin.

4. Use water that is close to body temperature—neither too hot nor too cold—to avoid increasing toxin absorption.

Beware of Small Household Items Becoming Big Hazards

Many parents are careful to keep sharp objects like knives and scissors out of reach to prevent their children from getting cut or injured. However, a commonly overlooked detail is the type of cups and bowls used in the house. Many families use glass cups and ceramic bowls, but if these fall and shatter, they can easily injure a child. We've encountered numerous cases where children were rushed to emergency rooms after being cut by broken glass. For safety, it's best for parents to give their children stainless steel cups and bowls, which won't shatter if dropped.

It's also important to warn children about the dangers of smaller items like chopsticks and toothpicks. These objects should never be used as toys, as a child could accidentally injure their eyes, which can have serious consequences.

Parents should also supervise children during

play, especially boys who often enjoy pretending to "fight" with toy weapons, which can quickly escalate into accidents. Children love to run, jump, and climb, which increases the risk of falls and injuries. This is especially true during physical activities, such as gym class, where following the teacher's instructions and observing proper safety rules are crucial.

Electrical Hazards at Home

Small household appliances, like power strips, can also pose risks. Power strips are a common electrical hazard in homes with children. Parents should secure them in areas out of reach or out of sight and ensure they are kept away from water. It's also important to replace old or worn power strips and avoid using them beyond their intended lifespan. Unplugging power strips when not in use is a good safety practice.

What should parents do if their child is electrocuted?
The first and most important step is to disconnect the child from the power source. Never pull the child away with your hands, as

this will only cause the rescuer to be electrocuted as well. There are many reports of entire families being electrocuted one after another because each person tried to pull the previous one off the source.

If a child is electrocuted, do not reach out with your hands, no matter how urgent the situation feels. Instead, use the most straightforward method—turn off the power at the circuit breaker. Most homes today have a circuit breaker or fuse box. Parents should run to the breaker and turn off all the switches. Once the power is cut, the child will automatically be disconnected from the source, and it will then be safe to move the child away.

If it's impossible to reach the breaker, use insulating objects like a dry wooden stick, board, rope, or cloth to separate the child from the electricity. Once the child is clear of the source, check their condition immediately.

With household electricity, there are usually two outcomes:
1. The child feels a brief electric shock and is

unharmed.

2. The child experiences cardiac arrest and loses consciousness.

If the child seems fine, that's the best possible outcome. However, parents should still observe the child closely for the next 24–48 hours, as delayed reactions, such as cardiac arrest, can occur. Some children may appear normal after an electric shock but might feel dizzy or have heart palpitations later, which could indicate heart damage. In such cases, take the child to the hospital immediately for a thorough check-up.

If the child's heart stops, perform CPR immediately while calling for emergency services. One critical point to remember is that some children may appear to be in a state of "apparent death" after electrocution, where both the heart and breathing are extremely weak. The child may stop breathing but still have a heartbeat, or vice versa. In rare cases, both breathing and the heartbeat may be weak but present. In these situations, don't give up on the child, even if they appear lifeless. There is also the possibility of the child's body becoming rigid, but this doesn't mean the child is deceased; CPR should still be attempted. In rare cases, electrical burns may occur, and the child should be taken to a hospital with a burn unit.

Toxic Plants at Home

Many people enjoy keeping plants in their homes, but if you have children, be cautious. Some plants contain substances that can have harmful effects if inhaled by pregnant women or children. Avoid keeping plants like daffodils, mimosa, oleander, tulips, and poinsettias, as they may contain toxins harmful to children.

Toys to Be Cautious Of

Based on experience and research, here are 10 types of toys that pose a higher risk to children. Parents should either avoid giving these toys to children or ensure they are played with under supervision:

1. Projectile toys, such as toy guns with bullets,

which can cause serious injuries.

2. Toys with strings, like yo-yos, which can wrap around a child's fingers or neck, leading to tissue death or suffocation.

3. Masks, which can cause oxygen deprivation, leading to dizziness or fainting if worn for too long.

4. Balloons, which can burst and injure a child. Hydrogen balloons, in particular, are prone to dangerous explosions.

5. Small toys, like building blocks, which can be accidentally swallowed and become airway obstructions.

6. Metal toys, which may contain toxic lead.

7. Sharp-edged toys, which can easily cut or injure a child.

8. Toy vehicles, which can lead to falls and injuries.

9. Musical toys, as low-quality sounds can damage a child's hearing.

10. Stuffed animals, which can harbor dust and allergens, leading to respiratory issues like coughing, asthma, or even skin rashes in sensitive children.

Keep Children Within Sight During Travel

Many families now own cars and often take road trips together. However, I'd like to remind everyone: never leave a child alone in the car after parking.

Emergency Scene

I once encountered a situation where a young couple parked their car by the roadside without turning off the engine and left their child inside while they went into a small shop. The child started playing and accidentally pressed the automatic window button while sticking their head out of the window. The window rolled up and trapped the child's head. Fortunately, two passersby intervened and managed to lower the window, freeing the child. When the parents returned, they found their child crying non-stop, likely from pain or fright. Concerned, they called emergency services, and we arrived to examine the child. Fortunately, there were no serious issues. The child was incredibly lucky; without the quick actions of those passersby, the outcome could have been tragic.

Some people believe that automatic car windows should reverse when they detect an obstruction. However, you shouldn't rely on this feature. I've seen tests conducted by TV stations using objects like celery and cucumbers to check this function, and many cars don't have it. Worse, some car windows are very sharp and can quickly sever objects caught in them. There have even been reports of children dying from being trapped by car windows—parents must be vigilant.

Additionally, never lock your child in a parked car with the engine off. Cars are enclosed spaces, and the oxygen level inside will deplete quickly. In hot weather, the temperature inside can rise rapidly, leading to heatstroke, unconsciousness, or even death.

Car Safety for Children
There are other essential safety concerns when

driving with children:

1. Never hold a child on your lap while sitting in a car seat. A child weighing 16 kg (about 35 lbs) in a car traveling at 70 km/h (43 mph) is equivalent to a 280 kg (617 lb) object. In a collision, it's nearly impossible to hold onto the child, and they are usually the first to be thrown forward, risking severe injury to the neck or spine.

2. Never allow a child to use an adult seatbelt while sitting in the front passenger seat. In the event of a crash, the belt can injure the child's neck or cause suffocation.

3. Don't allow children to move around freely in the back seat. In a side collision or sudden stop, they could be thrown from the vehicle.

The correct way to secure a child is to use an appropriate child safety seat installed in the back seat. If the child is under four years old, the seat should be rear-facing. Older children can use a forward-facing seat.

Keep an Eye on Your Child Outdoors

When taking children on trips, parents must keep a close eye on them to prevent accidents.

Emergency Scene

On one occasion, a family took their child on a nature outing. The child, full of energy, wandered off and climbed a tree. In just two minutes of the parents being distracted, the child fell from the tree and fractured their forearm, crying in pain. Luckily, someone nearby had first-aid training and was able to stabilize the injury before the child was taken to the emergency center.

Key Reminder: When a child suffers a fracture, never attempt to reset the bone yourself. Doing so could cause further damage. Instead, immobilize the limb using any materials at hand and take the child to the hospital immediately for proper treatment. Additionally, children's bones are not fully developed and are prone to dislocation. Sometimes simple activities, such as an adult pulling the child up or down stairs or helping them get dressed, can result in a condition called "nursemaid's elbow" (radial head subluxation). While it may seem easy for doctors to pop the joint back in place, this requires skill. Parents should never attempt to do this themselves.

What to Do if a Child Knocks Out a Tooth
When children play outdoors, they might trip and injure their teeth, possibly knocking one out. If this happens, it's crucial to find the tooth as soon as possible to maximize the chances of successful reimplantation.

- Gently clean the tooth if it's dirty, using saline solution. Hold the tooth by the crown, not the root, and avoid rubbing or wiping the root, as this can damage the periodontal ligament tissue.
- Do not wrap the tooth in paper or dry cloth, as this can dry it out.
- Place the tooth back in its socket immediately if possible, and go to the hospital. If this isn't feasible, prevent the tooth from drying out by placing it in fresh cold milk, saline solution, or under the tongue (for older children or adults, not younger kids who may swallow it).

The success rate of reimplantation is over 90% if done within 30 minutes. After two hours, the success rate drops to less than 10%.

Key Travel Safety Tips

When traveling with children, never let them out of your sight, and don't allow them to wander too far. Hazards such as falls, electric shocks, drowning, snake or insect bites, and sprains are common in unfamiliar environments. If an accident does occur, refer to the first-aid techniques discussed earlier.

First Aid for Snake Bites: Apply a Tourniquet and Go to the Hospital Immediately

While traveling, parents must keep a close watch on their children. In addition to ensuring they don't stray too far, there is another critical situation to be aware of: children may get bitten by snakes hidden in grassy or bushy areas. Such incidents occur almost every year. Therefore, when taking children on trips, parents should not only choose safe routes but also be familiar with essential first aid measures for venomous snake bites.

How to Distinguish Between Venomous and Non-Venomous Snakes

Venomous snakes have two types of venom. One is hemotoxic, which primarily causes severe local symptoms, intense pain, and may lead to bleeding, kidney failure, and heart damage, eventually resulting in death. The other is neurotoxic, which causes milder local symptoms but more severe systemic effects, such as the child falling into a coma. Some venomous snakes have only one type of venom, while others have both.

If you are unable to determine whether the snake is venomous, treat the bite as if it is from a venomous snake. Even if you're sure it's not a venomous bite, do not take it lightly. You should still go to the hospital immediately for a tetanus antitoxin injection.

So, what should parents do if they find that their child has been bitten by a venomous snake?

Some readers might be thinking: "Wait a minute, Dr. Jia, I've seen on TV or read in books that there are many steps involved, like sucking out the venom with your mouth, cutting the wound, and other procedures. Why haven't you mentioned these?" It's not that I'm not mentioning them—those steps are unnecessary and may even worsen the injury.

According to the latest first aid guidelines, these measures provide very little benefit and may cause harm if not done correctly. For example, sucking out the venom, whether with your mouth or with a vacuum device, removes only a small amount of venom and may worsen the wound. If venom is sucked out with the mouth, the rescuer could even be poisoned. As for cutting the wound, most people cannot do this properly, and it increases the risk of infection. Squeezing the wound to expel the venom can easily promote the spread of toxins if done improperly. Therefore, it's better to stick to the basics—apply a tourniquet and rush the child to the hospital for professional treatment.

Apart from snake bites, bites from household pets are also common.

Many people enjoy keeping pets, such as dogs, cats, hamsters, and even turtles. For empty nesters, childless couples, or single individuals, having a pet can be a great emotional comfort. However, if there are children in the house, especially young ones, parents need to be vigilant. One careless moment and the child could be bitten or scratched. So what should you do in such cases?

If a child is bitten or scratched by a pet, parents should immediately rinse the wound thoroughly under running cool water for at least 20 minutes, using soapy water if possible. While rinsing, gently squeeze the area around the wound to help expel as much bacteria as possible. For thicker areas of skin, you can also use a cupping method to draw out bacteria before rinsing with running cool water again.

After rinsing the wound, disinfect it with alcohol, iodine, or povidone-iodine, as the wound may contain not only rabies virus but also bacteria such as tetanus. Do not bandage the wound or apply medication; instead, take the child to the hospital immediately. Regardless of whether the pet has been vaccinated against rabies, it is best to have the child receive a rabies vaccine after being bitten or scratched. Pets might carry the rabies virus even if they don't show symptoms. This is especially important if the child's skin was broken during the bite or scratch, as a rabies vaccine is critical to prevent potentially fatal consequences.

Although rabies is rare, once symptoms appear, the fatality rate is 100%. So, to be safe, always take your child to the hospital for a rabies shot after a pet bite.

Lastly, while it's fine to keep pets, parents must be aware of the potential harm they could pose to children. Also, ensure that pets are properly vaccinated, dewormed, bathed regularly, and have their nails trimmed. This is crucial for protecting both children and others.

Let's Learn New First Aid Skills: First Aid for Venomous Snake Bites
1. Have the child sit down and remain still, keeping the affected limb lowered. Movement can increase blood circulation and speed up the spread of venom.
2. Tie a tourniquet about 5 cm above the wound on the side closer to the heart, making sure it's tight enough to fit one finger underneath.
3. Rush the child to the hospital immediately and

seek professional medical help.

4. While on the way to the hospital, loosen the tourniquet every 30 minutes for one or two minutes each time.

Postscript

After much effort and perseverance, this book is finally about to be published.

Throughout my decades-long career in emergency care, I have treated countless patients and experienced many vivid and compelling cases. By sharing some of these stories, I hope to provide readers with both entertainment during their leisure time and thought-provoking insights. I also hope readers can gain some useful lessons and learn essential first aid knowledge.

To this day, I have worked in emergency medical care for a full 49 years, and I have been involved in public first aid education for 31 years. People call me "China's First Person in Public First Aid Education," which makes me feel a bit uneasy, as I know how limited an individual's strength is. At the same time, I am pleased to see that many like-minded doctor friends are also working tirelessly to promote medical knowledge. I sincerely hope that more of my colleagues will join in spreading medical knowledge and improving people's health.

I have been fortunate enough to dedicate my life to the field of emergency care, especially at the Beijing Emergency Medical Center. This work has enriched my life experiences, allowing me to witness the vastness of the world while also seeing the beauty and ugliness of humanity. For the sake of patients and for life itself, I have experienced successes and joys that most people will never know, as well as the frustration and sorrow of not being able to save a life, and the pain of being misunderstood.

I have been interviewed countless times by newspapers, magazines, TV stations, radio stations, and websites. One reporter once asked me, "Dr. Jia, have you ever had any regrets?" Without thinking, I responded, "I have grievances, but no regrets!" The reporter immediately slapped his thigh, exclaiming, "What a phrase—grievances, but no regrets!" Another reporter once wrote an article about me titled "The Chivalrous Doctor," and just the title alone moved me for a long time.

If there is a next life, I would still choose this noble profession, and I would still be honored to be part of the Beijing Emergency Medical Center team.

Today, most people spend time learning practical skills like computers and driving, but for the sake of ourselves, our loved ones, friends, and colleagues—for life itself—I hope more people will learn basic first aid knowledge and skills to be prepared for any emergency. Only when first aid knowledge is widespread will everyone have the chance to save lives and be saved.

The most precious thing in life is life itself, and we only get one.

I find it hard to part from the emergency care work that I love and have dedicated my life to. Even though I have retired and can no longer personally rescue patients, I can still continue to contribute to the health and lives of the Chinese people by spreading first aid awareness, concepts, knowledge, and skills to more people.

I hope that those who read this book will not only learn about the work and life of an emergency doctor but also gain some of the first aid knowledge and skills they need. That is my purpose in writing this book. It can also be used as a first aid textbook.

Due to time constraints and my limited expertise and writing ability, there may inevitably be some shortcomings in the book, and I hope readers will forgive them! I also hope that readers will provide valuable feedback to help improve it.